Anaesthetics for Junior Doctors and Allied Professionals

The essential guide

Edited by

DANIEL COTTLE

Consultant in Anaesthesia
Lancashire Teaching Hospitals NHS Foundation Trust

and

SHONDIPON LAHA

Consultant in Anaesthesia
Lancashire Teaching Hospitals NHS Foundation Trust

Foreword by

PETER NIGHTINGALE

MB BS, FRCA, FRCP, FFICM, FRCP Ed
Consultant in Anaesthesia & Intensive Care Medicine
University Hospital of South Manchester

Radcliffe Publishing

Radcliffe Publishing Ltd
33–41 Dallington Street
London
EC1V 0BB
United Kingdom

www.radcliffehealth.com

British Library Cataloguing in Publication Data

A catalogue record for this book is available from the British Library.

ISBN-13: 978 184619 551 8

The paper used for the text pages of this book
is FSC® certified. FSC (The Forest Stewardship
Council®) is an international network to promote
responsible management of the world's forests.

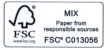

Typeset by Darkriver Design, Auckland, New Zealand
Printed and bound by TJI Digital, Padstow, Cornwall, UK

Contents

Foreword

When asked to write this foreword for *Anaesthesics for Junior Doctors and Allied Professionals* the thought crossed my mind as to why, in today's world of easy internet access, when access to information is just a few clicks away on a smartphone, do people still buy books such as this one? It was Samuel Johnson who said 'Knowledge is of two kinds. We know a subject ourselves, or we know where we can find information upon it.' This statement, and the title of the book, gives the answer. Beginners in any discipline need a template and didactic facts to start the process of achieving mastery in their field. In a little over 240 pages, this book, written by anaesthetists in daily active practice, distils the essence of what anaesthesia is about for neophytes and those who work with anaesthetists. It provides the basic background and ground rules for how anaesthetists work, how they approach a problem and how one can prepare for it. Some of the initial chapters could be usefully read by all surgeons, especially those in Foundation Training posts, and medical students considering an anaesthetic or intensive placement. The use of lists, key points and limited use of references help make the book easy to read, or dip into between cases, and keep it a manageable size whilst still providing a mine of information for the target audience – it's all in the title.

Peter Nightingale MB BS, FRCA, FRCP, FFICM, FRCP Ed
Consultant in Anaesthesia & Intensive Care Medicine
University Hospital of South Manchester
June 2013

Preface

Arriving in the anaesthetic room for the first time can be a daunting experience. You will be closely supervised, but everything will seem very new. Surgery is a stressful life-event for the patient and your job as an anaesthetist is to make it as safe and as comfortable as you can while ensuring the best outcome possible. As anaesthesia is induced and the patient becomes unconscious the patient entrusts his or her life to the anaesthetic team. As part of that team we must look after some of the patient's most basic functions that maintain life.

Anaesthesia is no longer the preserve of the medical anaesthetist. It increasingly features in undergraduate education and postgraduate programmes of the varied professions that care for our patients. Many of the competencies may have to be acquired in a short period of time, alongside the use of many new drugs and much new equipment.

There are many anaesthesia textbooks on the market. The majority detail the complicated physiology, pharmacology and physics required to gain a deep understanding of the subjects, to prepare for a consultant career and to pass the Fellowship of the Royal College of Anaesthetists exams.

This is not an exam preparation book, although it will provide a basis for the Fellowship of the Royal College of Anaesthetists Primary examination. This book is not just aimed at anaesthetists at the beginning of their career. We hope that Foundation trainees, Acute Care Common Stem trainees, Intensive Care Medicine trainees and medical students, operating department trainees and nurses also find it of benefit. It provides practical and clinically relevant advice in easily understandable sections that prepare the novice for his or her days in theatre. It will allow you to understand the most common drugs and it will provide a rationale for those we use.

The later chapters provide a quick, clinical reference for dealing with common problems and emergencies. We intentionally asked our own trainees to write the majority of chapters, and their advice is based on their own experiences.

Anaesthesia is a fascinating aspect of hospital practice. We hope that this book provides a little insight into the basics, especially for the many that spend only a few months experiencing this discipline.

Daniel Cottle
Shondipon Laha
June 2013

List of contributors

Claire Allen
Specialist Trainee
North West Deanery

Balsam Altemimi
Consultant in Anaesthesia
Aintree University Hospital NHS Trust

Nitin Arora
Consultant in Anaesthesia
Heart of England NHS Trust

Charlotte Ash
Specialist Trainee
North West Deanery

Kate Bailey
Specialist Trainee
North West Deanery

Steve Benington
Consultant in Anaesthesia
Central Manchester University Hospitals

Kailash Bhatia
Consultant in Anaesthesia
Central Manchester University Hospitals

Sophie Bishop
Consultant in Anaesthesia
University Hospital of South Manchester

Geraint Briggs
Consultant in Anaesthesia
University Hospital of South Manchester

Jess Briggs
Specialist Trainee
North West Deanery

Gillian Campbell
Specialist Trainee
North West Deanery

Katie Carden
Anaesthetic Practitioner
East Lancashire Hospitals Trust

Jasbir Chhabra
Consultant in Anaesthesia
Dudley Group of Hospitals NHS Trust

Natalie Cooper
Specialist Trainee
North West Deanery

Daniel Cottle
Consultant in Anaesthesia
Lancashire Teaching Hospitals NHS
   Foundation Trust

Anna Crosby
Specialist Trainee
North West Deanery

Leanne Darwin
Specialist Trainee
North West Deanery

Andrew Davies
Specialist Trainee
North West Deanery

Paul Dean
Consultant in Anaesthesia
East Lancashire Hospitals Trust

Nick Doree
Consultant in Anaesthesia
Wrightington, Wigan and Leigh NHS
  Foundation Trust

Tina Duff
Consultant in Anaesthesia
Central Manchester University Hospitals

Daniel Flaherty
Theatre Support Worker
East Lancashire Hospitals Trust

Peter Frank
Specialist Trainee
North West Deanery

Vandana Girotra
Specialist Trainee
North West Deanery

James Hanison
Specialist Trainee
North West Deanery

Shondipon Laha
Consultant in Anaesthesia
Lancashire Teaching Hospitals NHS
  Foundation Trust

Simon Maguire
Consultant in Anaesthesia
University Hospital of South Manchester

Kenneth McGrattan
Consultant in Anaesthesia
Lancashire Teaching Hospitals NHS
  Foundation Trust

Claire Moore
Consultant in Anaesthesia
University Hospital of South Manchester

John Moore
Consultant in Anaesthesia
Central Manchester University Hospitals

Daniel Nethercott
Consultant in Anaesthesia
Bolton NHS Foundation Trust

Ruth Nicholson
Operating Department Practitioner
East Lancashire Hospitals Trust

Justin Roberts
Specialist Trainee
North West Deanery

Cristian Salbaticu
Specialist Trainee
North West Deanery

Amanda Shaw
Consultant in Anaesthesia
Lancashire Teaching Hospitals NHS
  Foundation Trust

Nicola Smith
Specialist Trainee
North West Deanery

Craig Spencer
Consultant in Anaesthesia
Lancashire Teaching Hospitals NHS
  Foundation Trust

Matthew Stagg
Specialist Trainee
North West Deanery

Zara Townley
Specialist Trainee
North West Deanery

Fiona Wallace
Specialist Trainee
North West Deanery

Nick Wisely
Consultant in Anaesthesia
University Hospital of South Manchester

Acknowledgement

The figures are based on originals provided by Kelvin Pankhurst.

To Jen, thanks for all your support.
DC

To my parents and sister, Jonny, Ned, Meg
and my wife who all put up with me.
Thank you.
SL

CHAPTER 1

The fundamental principles of anaesthesia

DANIEL NETHERCOTT

Anaesthesia provides the vital interface between the surgeon and the patient. Implicit in a patient giving their consent to surgery is that they will be protected from the undesirable aspects of the experience by some form of anaesthesia, which can be:
- *regional* – where only a proportion of the body is rendered insensate
- *general* – in which consciousness is impaired
- or a combination of both.

Serious contemplation should be given when seeking to artificially diminish a person's consciousness, even temporarily and with their agreement. Consciousness is perhaps what defines the experience of being alive and although anaesthesia has become so common as to seem mundane, patients still entrust us with something fundamental, even profound.

THE ELEMENTS OF ANAESTHESIA

It is not always the case that patients want to be completely removed from the experience of their surgery. Some fear the loss of control and autonomy from allowing themselves to be made unconscious and so elect to have a regional technique alone. Other patients take interest in being able to watch a part of the procedure, such as an arthroscopy. Caesarean section under spinal anaesthesia is the default technique in most circumstances to allow the patient to fully experience and remember the birth. However, all patients need to be spared from pain, and surgeons require the operative site to be still and accessible. Therefore, a standard general anaesthetic can be broken down into the provision of three separate but interrelated elements: (1) *hypnosis*, (2) *analgesia* and (3) *akinesia*.

Hypnosis

Hypnosis means that the patient has no conscious awareness of the surgery taking place, nor any memory of what has happened after he or she wakes up.

Anaesthesia is not, of course, a binary state. There exists a continuum from:
- fully awake

- lightly sedated
- nicely asleep
- acceptably unrousable
- worryingly comatose
- to, eventually, irredeemable death: 'The undiscover'd country, from whose bourn no traveller returns.'[1]

These are referred to as *planes* of anaesthesia.

Processed electroencephalography such as the bispectral index monitor measures brain activity directly and can be interpreted as indicating depth of anaesthesia, but use of these monitors is not currently standard practice for most UK anaesthetists.

Analgesia

This means that the patient is not experiencing any pain or unpleasant sensations during the surgery. Pain is 'an unpleasant sensory and emotional experience associated with actual or potential tissue damage, or described in terms of such damage', and so it is subjective. Therefore, in reality it is not absolutely true to describe a patient who is unconscious as experiencing 'pain'. However, physiological responses mediated by the autonomic nervous system are commonly interpreted as signs of increased nociception (the neural process of encoding and processing noxious stimuli).

The end point for the use of analgesic techniques during general anaesthesia is therefore *autonomic stability*. An anaesthetised patient who is tachycardic and hypertensive with dilated pupils and beads of sweat on his or her forehead might be nicely managed with a generous intravenous dose of fentanyl.

Akinesia

Only the most generous and forgiving of surgeons allows the patient to move around the operating table without passing comment. During some surgery – for example, on the middle ear or around the brainstem – unexpected movement could cause disaster. Muscle relaxation can be important for surgical access, and increased tone in the abdominal muscles during laparotomy provides unnecessary opportunity for satirical remarks that are rarely becoming of trainee general surgeons.

BALANCED ANAESTHESIA

Modern techniques are built upon targeting these three elements with different drugs in different routes of administration to achieve a *balanced anaesthetic*. This refers to the use of specific agents for specific effects. To achieve akinesia and analgesia with a volatile agent alone (such as sevoflurane) would need such a high concentration that the side effects would start to cause trouble.

A judicious combination of anaesthetic agent, analgesic (or regional technique) and muscle relaxant will contribute all three required elements with minimal side effects. For example, a patient undergoing laparotomy could be successfully anaesthetised with an intravenous infusion of propofol and remifentanil, and intravenous bolus doses of atracurium. The patient could equally successfully be managed with inhaled sevoflurane, epidural infusion of bupivacaine and a continuous infusion of rocuronium.

It is a bit too simplistic to think of these three elements as being totally separate and solely achieved with different agents. Drugs delivered by various routes can interact in complex ways. For example, systemic opiates will contribute to overall depth of anaesthesia, and it is even postulated that muscle relaxants decrease afferent neural input associated with proprioception and might contribute to depth of anaesthesia too (although this would only be a small effect).[2]

THE ART OF ANAESTHESIA

Creating the right balance is where the *artistry* comes into it all, and where the frustrations begin for the novice who strives for competent, independent practice. Observing an experienced anaesthetist can give an illusion of simplicity and economy of action, and yet there can be quite a degree of individual variety in the approach to each case. With only a limited range of drugs and equipment to choose from, any two anaesthetists can manage the same case in different ways.

Although the 'recipe' might seem simple, success is often dependent on the skill and experience of the 'cook'. One element of this skill is being able to match the plane of anaesthesia to the degree of surgical stimulus. Some surgery only causes a little nociception and so a 'light' plane of anaesthesia is suitable. Some surgical events are enormously 'painful'/stimulating and the patient needs to be 'deepened' to counter this. Such differing needs can occur within a few minutes of each other. With experience of the surgery (and the surgeon) the anaesthetist can predict and anticipate these changes and titrate the plane of anaesthesia accordingly.

The drug dose that gives the right plane of anaesthesia with least side effects differs between a frail, elderly patient with severe co-morbidities and a boisterous youth with intoxicating habits. A keen grasp of physiology and pharmacology is the basis on which to develop a clinical intuition that gets the balance right for each case.

BIPLANES AND BUTLERS

The work of the anaesthetist has attracted some common analogies. Comparison with aircraft pilots has been made,[3] which seems acceptable in the similarity between the excitement of the take-off and the landing being interspersed by the sitting-down and interest in a monitor; expecting calm travel but being prepared to avert rapidly intruding disaster. However, this comparison fails when it is recognised that aeroplanes are designed to fly but patients are not designed to be anaesthetised; that an aeroplane with a misfiring engine and a rusty fuselage would not be chanced in the air; and that aeroplanes rarely have people hacking at the fuel lines midflight.

The anaesthetist has perhaps more satisfyingly been characterised as P. G. Wodehouse's sage butler Jeeves to the surgeon's Bertie Wooster, guiding his hapless master, encouraging him in his darker moments, restraining his excesses, holding unexpected calamities at bay (in Bertie's case these always seem to come in the shape of menacing maiden aunts[4]) and deferring personal glory for the greater goal.

THE MAGIC TRICK

To take a person who is conversant, breathing spontaneously with a stable heart and blood flow, to render that person unconscious, apnoeic with depressed cardiac function by the use of powerful and dangerous drugs, to rescue that person immediately from this iatrogenic state with instruments, oxygen and other powerful drugs, to hold that person in limbo for as long as necessary, then to put that same person back as they were – talking, breathing, comfortable, unaware of anything having happened at all – can feel like a rather brilliant and magical trick. Preparation, vigilance and anticipation are vital to pull off the trick of anaesthesia without harming the patient or allowing him or her to come to harm.

SUMMARY

Divinum sedare dolorem (it is divine to alleviate pain) reads the motto of the Royal College of Anaesthetists, *in somno securitas* (safe in sleep) reads that of the Association of Anaesthetists of Great Britain and Ireland. Alleviating pain, horror and distress is indeed worthy, and striving to do it safely is imperative.

Key points

- Balanced anaesthesia requires hypnosis, analgesia and akinesia.
- The balance of the different elements depends upon the patient, the surgery and the anaesthetist's personal experience.
- The planes of anaesthesia describe the depth of anaesthesia, from awake to deeply comatose.
- Your anaesthetic must alleviate pain, facilitate surgery and ensure the patient's safety.

REFERENCES

1. Shakespeare W. *Hamlet*. Act 3, scene 1.
2. Bonhomme V, Hans P. Muscle relaxation and depth of anaesthesia: where is the missing link? *Br J Anaesth*. 2007; **99**(4): 456–60.
3. Hutchinson G. Biggles FRCA. *Today's Anaesthetist*. 1998; **13**: 83–4.
4. Wodehouse PG. *Aunts Aren't Gentlemen*. London: Barrie & Jenkins; 1974.

CHAPTER 2

A very brief history of anaesthesia

DANIEL NETHERCOTT

The death rate directly attributable to a general anaesthetic provided in a modern environment by a trained anaesthetist approximates to an impressively small 1 in 250 000.[1] For many hundreds of years before the discovery of what would now be recognised as anaesthesia, mankind has used the analgesic and sedative properties of opium, alcohol, mandrake, henbane and other naturally occurring substances to lessen the pain and horror of surgical procedures. None of these approaches proved acceptably safe, in contrast to the remarkable safety profile of modern anaesthetic practice.

In understanding the contemporary science of anaesthesia it is worth considering a brief timeline of some important steps in the development of general and regional anaesthesia.[2,3]

GENERAL ANAESTHESIA

1795   Humphry Davy realises that inhaling nitrous oxide makes him giggle and feel dizzy.

1825   Charles Waterton demonstrates the naturally occurring muscle relaxant curare to paralyse and then mechanically ventilate a tracheostomised donkey. (The indigenous people of South America having used it for hundreds of years in the form of poison-tipped arrows for hunting.)

1842   Dr. William Clarke uses ether to perform a dental extraction in Rochester, New York. Two months later, Dr. Crawford Long uses ether to excise a neck cyst in Danielsville, Georgia.

1844   Gardner Colton administers nitrous oxide to dentist Horace Wells for a dental extraction. Wells is inspired to make a bellows to administer the gas, but is then humiliated when he demonstrates it at Massachusetts General Hospital and the patient screams with agony. Wells develops an unhealthy relationship with chloroform and later commits suicide.

1846   Boston dentist William Morton provides anaesthesia with ether for removal of a neck tumour. The demonstration is successful, his technique having been honed by practice on his pet dog. Two months later, surgeon Robert Liston, the 'fastest knife in the West End', amputates a leg under ether anaesthesia in London. He declares, 'This Yankee dodge, gentlemen, beats mesmerism hollow!'

1848   Deaths due to general anaesthesia are reported.

1853   John Snow, English physician and 'the father of anaesthesia', administers chloroform to Queen Victoria for the birth of Prince Leopold. The Queen's approval softens the moral and medical opposition to anaesthesia for childbirth.

1872   Pierre-Cyprien Oré uses chloral hydrate for intravenous anaesthesia.

1912   Arthur Lawen, a German surgeon, uses curare in anaesthesia.

1913   Chevalier Jackson, an American laryngologist, uses a laryngoscope to intubate the trachea.

1937   Robert Macintosh becomes the first British professor of anaesthesia.

1942   Harold Griffith, Canadian anaesthetist, popularises the use of curare in anaesthesia.

1946   Curtis Mendelson, an American obstetrician, describes a syndrome of bronchopulmonary aspiration of stomach contents in obstetric general anaesthesia.

1948   The Faculty of Anaesthetists is established within the Royal College of Surgeons of England.

1950   The pharmacological properties of succinylcholine are discovered. Apocryphal stories abound of 'The Suxamethonium Run', whereby trainee anaesthetists intubate colleagues after they have self-injected the drug and then run as far as possible before paralysis.

1992   The (now independent) College of Anaesthetists is given Royal charter.

2007   The Faculty of Pain Medicine is formed within the Royal College of Anaesthetists.

2010   The Faculty of Intensive Care Medicine is formed with the Royal College of Anaesthetists and with the support of several of the other medical Royal Colleges.

REGIONAL ANAESTHESIA

1859   Cocaine is isolated by Friedrich Gaedcke, a German chemist.

1884   Before Sigmund Freud gains his famous interest in the sexual preoccupations of hysterical women, he enjoys the uplifting properties of cocaine and mentions its numbing effect to his friend Karl Koller. Koller demonstrates this effect publicly by sticking pins into his own eyes and then more sensibly uses it as a local anaesthetic for eye surgery.

1885   James Corning, an American neurologist, uses cocaine for spinal anaesthesia. August Bier, a German surgeon, later demonstrates it on himself, and describes the 'post-dural puncture headache'.

1901   Nicolae Racoviceanu-Piteşti, Romanian surgeon, reports providing analgesia with intrathecal opiates.

1902   Heinrich Braun, a German surgeon, describes the addition of adrenaline to local anaesthetic solutions to prolong the duration of action.

1908   August Bier introduces intravenous regional anaesthesia using procaine.

1943   Lidocaine is synthesised.

1945   Edward Tuohy, an American anaesthetist, popularises use of the 'Tuohy' needle for continuous spinal anaesthesia, although dentist Ralph Huber initially invented it.

1998   Intralipid is postulated as a treatment for local anaesthetic toxicity after success in an animal model.

SUMMARY

Anaesthesia has not developed as an end in itself but, rather, for the purpose of allowing surgical procedures to take place. The development of anaesthesia has allowed major advances in surgery, and surgical techniques and ambition have driven advances in anaesthesia. Developments in pharmacology, monitoring, equipment, training and resuscitation have made anaesthesia progressively safer for a wider range of patients.

REFERENCES

1. www.rcoa.ac.uk
2. Porter R. *The Greatest Benefit to Mankind: a medical history of humanity from antiquity to the present.* London: Harper Collins; 1997.
3. Yentis S, Hirsch N, Smith G. *Anaesthesia and Intensive Care A–Z: an encyclopaedia of principles and practice.* London: Butterworth-Heinemann; 2004.

CHAPTER 3

The anaesthetic day

DANIEL COTTLE

The anaesthetist's day differs from other specialities in the hospital for several reasons:
- you don't work on a ward
- you don't work in a firm
- you don't have any inpatients
- you'll spend most of your day using equipment
- there is a fair chance that some of your patients won't even be ill.

When you're new to anaesthetics you are supernumary, but don't rest on your laurels. This is a chance to use all those transferable skills that you didn't even know you had and to build an armoury of new ones. With good planning, careful management and plenty of communication everything should go well and you should certainly look good! The following section is an overview of the anaesthetist's working day with tips on how to make it easier. The details of anaesthesia are covered later.

THE NIGHT BEFORE
Forewarned is forearmed. Everything can move very fast in the morning, and if you don't know anything else about anaesthesia, then you should know about your patients.

Check the rota
- Which theatre you are working in?
- What type of surgery is it?
- Who are you going to be working with?

Get a copy of the operating list
- How you do this will differ depending on the department you are working in.
- Most departments will have theatre management software. This will allow you to access your lists in advance.
- If this (or more likely the password) is not available then ask the theatre receptionist for a copy.

Speak to the consultant or trainee who will supervise you

- Discuss what you already know.
- Explain what your training needs are.
- Arrange where and when to meet in the morning before your preoperative visits.
- It may be that the consultant already knows the patients and can tell you about them.

Go to see your patients

- Some patients are admitted the night before surgery, but most of your patients will have their operations as day cases.
- However, patients having major surgery or those who have complicated past medical histories may be brought in early.
- These patients can take a long time to assess, and while you aren't expected to provide them with a plan you should know all about their history before they arrive in the anaesthetic room.

THE MORNING OF SURGERY

The basics

- While you are no doubt thinking of the technical aspects of the day ahead, think of some of the little things first.
- You might think that you are going to get a locker, but most likely you aren't, so bring a bag that can store your valuables and paperwork.
- Some departments have freshly clean shoes to wear, but most don't. That means braving the 'random old shoes' in the changing room, which might turn out to be the consultant surgeon's. Avoid all this by buying some clean white trainers that you can store in your own box with your name on.
- You won't get that long for lunch and you don't want to spend it getting changed and walking to a canteen miles away. Always bring your own lunch, coffee and mug.

Assess your patients

- Most patients will have arrived that morning.
- If you know nothing about anaesthesia then at least you will have met your patients, have learned why they are there and what medical problems they might have.
- Try to see the patients with your consultant – it's a better learning experience and it will avoid those difficult questions you can't answer.

WHO IS WHO?

The operating department practitioner or anaesthetic nurse

- Whichever type of assistant you are working with they will perform the same job.
- An operating department practitioner (ODP) has trained as a practitioner in theatres and has rotated through scrub, anaesthetics and recovery.
- An anaesthetic nurse has gone through the standard nurse training and has then specialised in anaesthesia, and often in recovery as well.

- Learn the assistant's name and strike up a good working relationship. Make your first impression count.

There will also be the scrub nurse, who will prepare equipment and assist the surgeon. The scrub nurse will be supported by a runner – the runner may be a nurse or a healthcare assistant. Each theatre will have a sister or charge nurse in charge of the theatre and there will be more senior nurses coordinating the whole theatre suite.

SETTING UP THE ANAESTHETIC ROOM

Your ODP or anaesthetic nurse will have set up the anaesthetic room, but it is the anaesthetist's responsibility to check that everything has been done. Using and checking the equipment is covered in more detail later, but you should check the anaesthetic machines, suction units, all monitors and the airway equipment before the list starts. You should make sure that anything that you plan to use is present or available. Next, you should draw up your emergency drugs and anaesthesia. Your choice of drugs will depend on the anaesthesia required. Request intravenous lines to be run through and sign for the controlled drugs that you have used.

TEAM BRIEFING

Before each list begins, all members of the anaesthetic, surgical and scrub teams should meet to have a team briefing. This is an opportunity to be introduced to everyone, begin to build a rapport with the surgeon and get answers to any practical questions you may have. The running order of the list should be confirmed and any unexpected steps should be discussed.

Find out what position the surgeon wants; confirm *exactly* what the operation entails, what type of incision is expected and how long each case will take. This allows for a smoother running list and it allows you to plan positioning, intravenous lines, warming and post-operative analgesia. All hospitals now use World Health Organization checklists to confirm patient details, site of surgery and any expected problems.

On returning to the anaesthetic room you should have a similar detailed discussion with your ODP about your anaesthetic plan and what equipment you require. The consultant will do this initially, but it is an important aspect of making sure the patient is kept safe and you will be expected to contribute to this.

MANAGING A LIST

As well as anaesthetising patients you will be required to manage the list. Managing a list is a formal way of saying, 'keeping the list running efficiently and safely'. This will become even more important if it is the emergency list.

It will be your job to make sure that the patients are ready for theatre and that the ward staff receives the correct instructions. If there are any problems on the ward before the patient comes to theatre then the ward queries will most likely be directed to you.

Once the list is underway you should instruct the staff to send for the next patient. How soon you do this will depend on the hospital that you work in, how far away your patients are and whether there is a theatre reception. You should also keep good lines of communication open with the surgeons and the scrub staff if the order of the list is to be changed. Remember that other people might have pressures that you haven't considered.

AT THE END OF THE LIST

The end of the list means that it is time to relax after a hard day's work. In order to go home safe in the knowledge that all has been done there are a few last points that should be considered.

Go to see your patients

At the end of the list, try to make time to see all your patients (although if there have been no problems several of them will have gone home). This is the best way to get feedback about what works and what doesn't. Specifically enquire about pain, nausea and vomiting, sore throat and ability to eat and drink. In sicker patients, check their fluid balance. If there aren't any problems it will remind the patient of the young anaesthetist who helped that to happen!

Hand over your post-operative plan

If your patient is staying on the ward, ensure that those who need to be are aware of your plan and that you have anticipated likely problems. This may mean ward nurses and doctors, the critical care or outreach teams, the acute pain nurse, physiotherapists and the patient's family.

Clean up after yourself

Make sure that you have tidied away your leftover drugs and any sharps. You are personally responsible for the disposal of any controlled drugs not given to the patient. Also think about coffee mugs and other mess. Not doing this will guarantee a gradual erosion of your relationship with the anaesthetic staff.

Ensure that the controlled drug book has been signed

It can be very time-consuming for people to have to track you down later to sign the controlled dug book.

Remember to plan for the next day

Have you got your list? Who are you working with? Are any of the patients on the ward now?

Finally, remember to enjoy yourself!

Key points
- You are going to be entering a new environment and working in a different team structure. You will have to adapt your current practice.
- Be prepared the night before. Know as much as you can about the theatre list before you start it.
- Always see all of the patients on the list before surgery.
- Take part in the team briefing and know who everyone is in theatre.
- End the day by visiting your patients. Ensure that they comfortable and safe and get valuable feedback.

CHAPTER 4

Preoperative assessment and investigations

DANIEL COTTLE AND JAMES HANISON

An anaesthetist should see all patients before surgery. Some patients will also have been seen in a preoperative clinic, by either a specialist nurse or an anaesthetist, and had investigations and optimisation of medical conditions. Some conditions are considered in more detail in the special circumstances chapters.

The aims of your preoperative visit are:
- to introduce yourself and establish a rapport with the patient
- to take a history and examination
- to order or check relevant investigations
- if the patient has already been seen in the preoperative assessment clinic then the accuracy of the information should be checked and any changes noted
- to ensure that the patient understands the anaesthetic plan and still consents to surgery
- to answer any questions and attend to the emotional needs of your patient
- to ensure availability of cross-matched blood and critical care beds, if required.

HISTORY
This should tell you:
- specific information about previous anaesthesia
- information to plan practical aspects of the patient's anaesthetic
- a summary of medical diagnoses and previous surgery
- if the patient has any undiagnosed illness
- what risk the surgery poses for the patient.

Anaesthetic history
- What types of surgery and anaesthesia has the patient had, and when did he or she have them?
- Did the patient suffer any complications?
  > post-operative nausea and vomiting
  > airway difficulties
  > uncontrolled pain, failed regional anaesthesia

- › struggling to wake up
- › neuropraxia
- › dural puncture headache.
- Does the patient have any allergies?
- Is there a family history of problems under anaesthesia that could be hereditary?
  - › drug reactions
  - › malignant hyperthermia
  - › suxamethonium apnoea.
- Does the patient suffer from regular gastro-oesophageal reflux that rises up to the larynx, especially when lying flat? If so, then he or she will require intubation with a rapid sequence induction.
- Smoking, alcohol and illegal drug use?
- Loose teeth, caps, crowns, veneers or dentures?
- When did the patient last eat and drink?
- Height and weight (for drug dosing and infusion pumps).

The following is a list of systems that you should enquire about. More details can be found in the special circumstances section.

Cardiac disease

- Does the patient have critical ischaemia that requires intervention before surgery? (Only a very small number of patients do.)
- If the patient has ischaemic heart disease or left ventricular failure, how does it limit him or her and how will it effect your management?
- Enquire about previous cardiac interventions and medications.
- Does the patient require further investigations and interventions?
- What drugs should be stopped and which continued? In particular, aspirin, clopidogrel and warfarin (*see* Chapter 22).
- Will the patient require invasive monitoring?

Vascular disease

- Peripheral vascular disease is a strong indicator of ischaemic heart disease. Beware of asymptomatic patients who do not undertake any physical activity.
- The patient may require careful blood pressure control. Does the patient require invasive monitoring?
- These patients are often in poor health and have multiple co-morbidities that you should be aware of.

Respiratory disease

- Is the patient's disease stable and can it be optimised?
- How could the planned surgery or anaesthesia worsen the patient's respiratory function?
- Maximise treatment and ensure compliance with medication.
- Treat infection before going ahead with surgery.
- Is the patient a carbon dioxide retainer?
- Will the patient require post-operative oxygen?
- Can the surgery be performed under regional or local anaesthetic?

- Children with coughs and colds without fever and new respiratory signs should not have their surgery postponed.

Hypertension

- This is not an independent risk factor for post-operative morbidity and mortality, and white coat hypertension should not delay surgery. Don't alarm the patient. Allow the patient time to relax and repeat the measurement.
- End-organ damage such as heart failure and renal failure are risk factors and so their treatment should be optimised.
- If the patient and his or her general practitioner state that the patient's blood pressure is normally well controlled then surgery should proceed.

Diabetes mellitus

- What type is it and is the patient diet, tablet or insulin controlled?
- The perioperative control of diabetes will depend on the type of diabetes and the surgery (*see* Box 4.1). Ensure that you follow local guidelines.

BOX 4.1 The perioperative treatment of diabetes

Type 1 diabetes
- Ensure that the patient is starved for the shortest time possible. Withold the patient's normal insulin whilst starved.
- For afternoon surgery, allow breakfast 6 hours before with the patient's normal insulin dose.
- For short procedures and day case surgery, monitor the patient's blood sugars hourly. Feed at the next mealtime after surgery and administer the patient's normal insulin.
- For major surgery and prolonged starvation, an insulin sliding scale with dextro-saline and potassium infusion will be needed.

Type 2 diabetes requiring insulin
- Withhold oral antiglycaemics on the morning of surgery.
- Manage insulin as per type 1 diabetes.
- Restart oral antiglycaemics when a regular diet has been established.
- Consider a sliding scale for major surgery and prolonged starvation.

Type 2 diabetes on oral antiglycaemics
- Ensure that the patient is starved for the shortest time possible. Give breakfast on the morning of afternoon surgery with the patient's normal medication.
- Withhold oral antiglycaemics before surgery.
- For short procedures and day case surgery, monitor the patient's blood sugars hourly. Feed at the next mealtime after surgery and administer the patient's normal medication.

Patients with diet-controlled type 2 diabetes can be managed like non-diabetic patients. Treat hypoglycaemia promptly with oral or intravenous glucose.

- You will need to prevent hypoglycaemia and ketoacidosis.
- Enquire about end-organ damage – particularly, heart failure, renal failure and autonomic dysfunction.

Endocrine

- Is the patient's treatment optimal and how will it continue throughout the perioperative period, particularly if the patient is to be nil by mouth?
- Patients who have taken prednisolone 10 mg daily for longer than 3 months will require hydrocortisone 25 mg at induction. Hydrocortisone 100 mg/day is required for moderate and major surgery.

Nephrology

- Is the patient's renal failure stable and what are his or her electrolytes?
- What is the patient's fluid balance status?
- Does the patient require dialysis and how will this be arranged perioperatively?

Rheumatology

- Rheumatological diseases affect multiple systems and can have a large influence on your anaesthetic.
- Look for difficult airways, a fixed neck or neck instability.
- Will arthritis or spondylitis make neuroaxial anaesthesia difficult?
- Also consider lung fibrosis, renal failure and steroid use.

Neurology

- Neurological deficit should be documented before anaesthesia to allow accurate assessment and comparison later.
- Epilepsy should be well controlled and the patient compliant with his or her anti-epileptic medication. The patient's anti-epileptic medication needs to be continued perioperatively.
- Bulbar weakness is a high risk for aspiration.
- Neurological injury, raised intracranial pressure, myasthenia gravis and myotonic dystrophy require specialist care.

Functional capacity

- If a patient can walk up a flight of stairs without stopping (4 METs) without cardiorespiratory symptoms, then he or she should be able to proceed to anaesthesia.

EXAMINATION

Not all patients will require a full examination but all should have had their heart and lungs auscultated before going to theatre.

Your examination should follow the standard for all medical examinations but you may need to concentrate on some specific aspects.

From the end of the bed

- Pallor and anaemia
- The patient's weight and distribution of adipose tissue

- Cachexia
- Smoking and high alcohol intake

Airway assessment
See Chapter 9.

Cardiovascular
- Prolonged capillary refill indicates low cardiac output or deficient fluid balance
- Pulse rate and volume and the presence of ectopic beats
- Raised jugular venous pressure, hepato-jugular reflex, displaced apex beat and a third heart sound indicate heart failure
- The presence of new murmurs should be investigated further

Respiratory
- Tar staining indicates high cigarette intake
- Blue bloater or pink puffer?
- Cough with production of sputum
- Respiratory rate and oxygen saturations on air as a baseline in patients with respiratory failure
- Assess chest expansion – is there abdominal splinting of the diaphragm?
- Percuss and auscultate the chest

Abdominal
- If indicated by the history
- Does a heavy drinker have the stigmata of chronic liver disease?

Vascular access
- Are peripheral veins visible or palpable? (Try to avoid the anticubital fossa, as flexing the arm will prevent fluid flow)
- Does the patient need local anaesthetic cream?
- Are the central venous sites accessible?
- Does the patient have a good radial pulse for an arterial line?

Regional anaesthesia
- Will you be able to perform a neuroaxial block?
- Can you identify the bony landmarks of the spine and will the patient be able to adopt the necessary position?
- Are other sites for nerve blocks accessible?
- Is the site free from local infection?

INVESTIGATIONS
The National Institute for Health and Clinical Excellence[1] has produced guidance for ordering preoperative investigations. This prevents unnecessary investigations being ordered and prevents delaying surgery because the correct ones haven't been done. The Association of Anaesthetists of Great Britain and Ireland have adopted these guidelines.[2]

Patients who have been to the preoperative assessment clinic should have had the necessary investigations ordered and checked. You should check them yourself.

Avoid ordering additional tests, which won't actually change your anaesthetic practice. Patients who are ASA 1–2 (American Society of Anesthesiologists Classification 1–2), undergoing surgery grades 1–2 do not require routine investigations.

Bedside tests

Pulse oximetry and non-invasive blood pressure analysers are cheap, reliable and almost omnipresent in the modern-day hospital. Every patient for every procedure should have had a record of the following measurements prior to surgery:

- heart rate
- SpO_2 (percentage saturation of haemoglobin with oxygen)
- blood pressure.

Blood tests

Full blood count

- Haemoglobin levels, white blood cell counts (including differential counts) and platelet counts are provided. The haemoglobin should be greater than 10 mg/dL for moderate or major surgery. A new diagnosis of anaemia should be referred for investigation. Raised white cells indicate infection and source should be sought. Platelets should be greater than 100×10^9/dL.

Renal function

- The urea and electrolytes test – sodium and potassium levels are provided and these are essential for every cell in the body. Abnormalities in these electrolytes may require further investigation. The probable cause, the severity of the derangement and the urgency of the surgery will determine if surgery needs to be delayed.
- Urea and creatinine levels are provided to assist in evaluating renal function.

Coagulation profile

- Prothrombin time and international normalised ratio assess the extrinsic clotting system. One of the uses of this test is to assess anticoagulation with warfarin.
- Activated partial thromboplastin time assesses the intrinsic clotting system in the blood. This is most commonly affected by anticoagulation with unfractionated heparin.
- Platelet inhibiting agents such as aspirin and clopidogrel will prolong bleeding without affecting the prothrombin time and activated partial thromboplastin time values.
- The efficacy of low-molecular-weight heparin is assessed using the activated factor 10 assay. This is not required prior to surgery.

Random serum glucose

- Random serum glucose measures the concentration of glucose in the blood of a non-fasted patient. Levels should not exceed 7.8 mmol/L. Levels higher than this suggest impaired glucose tolerance or diabetes and warrant further investigation.

Arterial blood gas analysis

● Arterial blood gas analysis will give levels of dissolved gases in the blood (oxygen, pO_2; carbon dioxide, pCO_2) and an evaluation of the acid-base status of the blood (pH, bicarbonate and base excess).
● Some analysers will also give sodium, potassium, chloride, haematocrit and lactate. These make arterial blood gases useful during major surgery.

Sickle cell testing

● Sickle cell testing is recommended preoperatively in all patients from the following ethnic groups: North African, West African, South/sub–Saharan African and Afro-Caribbean. Surgery can provoke a sickle crisis.
● Diagnosis of sickle cell trait or disease would have future implications for the patient and this should be discussed prior to testing.
● Patients with sickle cell disease should have their surgery in a specialist centre.

Pregnancy testing

● This test is essential in any woman who has a risk of being pregnant.
● Beta human chorionic gonadotrophin levels are elevated in pregnancy and can be tested from urine or blood. If there is a high index of suspicion the test should still be done on women that are on regular contraception or have had recent menstruation.
● Patients should always be counselled prior to pregnancy testing.

Urinalysis

Modern urine dipstick kits can detect protein, pH, ketones, glucose, red blood cells, white blood cells and specific gravity. Diseases of the renal tract and systemic diseases such as diabetes may be detected.

Electrocardiogram

The electrocardiogram (ECG) is another bedside test that is quick and simple to perform in the modern hospital setting. Patients with risk factors for ischaemic cardiac disease should be screened with this test.[2] It also detects conduction and electrolyte abnormalities that may be life-threatening under anaesthesia if not detected prior to surgery.

Chest X-ray

Chest X-rays are not part of preoperative health screening. They should only be used to answer specific questions (e.g. to check the position of pacemaker leads).

Lung function tests

● Peak expiratory flow rate is a bedside test that evaluates the peak flow (in litres per minute) on a single maximal expiratory effort following a period of deep inspiration. The test may be repeated to determine reproducibility.
● It measures obstruction to flow and is an objective test of obstructive lung disease (asthma, chronic obstructive pulmonary disease).
● Spirometry testing provides more information, specifically FEV_1 (forced expiratory volume over 1 second) and FVC (forced vital capacity), both of

which are used to determine severity of disease in chronic conditions such as chronic obstructive pulmonary disease and lung fibrosis. The test requires more specialised equipment and more skilled operators to generate and analyse the results.

Echocardiography
- This technique utilises ultrasound technology and Doppler calculations to produce two-dimensional images of the heart and analyse flow.
- It may be performed via the transthoracic or the transoesophageal route (the transoesophageal route provides more data but it is more invasive).
- This test requires skilled staff to perform and analyse the test. Commonly reported data includes:
  › visualisation of the atria, ventricles and valves of the heart
  › evidence of stenosis or regurgitation of valves and pressure gradients across the valves
  › systolic and diastolic function of the ventricles, including the left ventricular ejection fraction.

CARDIOPULMONARY EXERCISE TESTING
Cardiopulmonary exercise testing (CPEX) is a well-established tool that has been used outside of the hospital setting (such as sports medicine) for many years. The test measures the cardiovascular and respiratory reserves of the patient; reserves that are required in the post-operative period to recover from the acute surgical insult. There is increasing use of CPEX preoperatively, and many patients undergoing surgical procedures associated with a high mortality undergo the test.

The test comprises several components, as follows.
- The patient is exposed to an increasing ramp of exercise. This may be performed on a cycle ergometer or a treadmill. The exercise time is usually 10 minutes.
- Continuous ECG monitoring is undertaken. This exercise ECG subtracts artefact and detects ST segment abnormalities during the test that indicate exercise-induced myocardial ischaemia.
- Non-invasive blood pressure monitoring.
- The patient's inspiratory and expiratory gases are measured via a mouthpiece and nose clip or tightly fitting mask. This allows measurement of the:
  › rate of oxygen consumption (VO_2)
  › rate of CO_2 production (VCO_2).[3]

As the patient undergoes increasing levels of exercise, his or her tissues initially undergo *aerobic* metabolism. The VO_2 and the VCO_2 both increase linearly and at the same rate of increase. This reflects increasing tissue oxygen demand that is being met by an increasing oxygen delivery.
- As the exercise continues to increase, a point is reached where the cardiorespiratory system cannot provide oxygenated blood to the tissues at the rate required to meet their oxygen demand.
- This point is termed the *anaerobic threshold* and it can be measured during CPEX by the point at which the rate of increase of VCO_2 outstrips the rate of increase of VO_2.

- This reflects anaerobic metabolism exceeding aerobic metabolism and the accumulation of lactate in tissues.
- An anaerobic threshold less than 11 mL/minute/kg is associated with a poor outcome post-operatively.
- CPEX results are usually combined with other risk indicators to determine surgical risk.

A poor outcome in CPEX can be used to:
- counsel patients of risk of surgery preoperatively
- plan for higher levels of care post-operatively (high dependency unit and intensive care unit care)
- consider non-surgical management options.

TABLE 4.1 The Association of Anaesthetists of Great Britain and Ireland[2] guidelines adopted from the National Institute for Health and Clinical Excellence[1]

Test	Indication
Electrocardiogram	Age >80 years
	Age >60 years, surgery grade ≥3
	Cardiovascular disease
	Severe renal disease
Full blood count	Age >60 years and surgery grade ≥2
	Adults for surgery grade ≥3
	Severe renal disease
Urea and electrolytes	Age ≥60 years and surgery grade ≥3
	All surgery grades ≥4
	All renal disease
	Severe cardiovascular disease
Pregnancy test	Women who may be pregnant
Sickle cell	Family history or racial history
Chest X-ray	Patients requiring critical care

Only order additional tests if the patient's co-morbidities require them. Patients who you think require echocardiography, CPEX testing or myocardial perfusion scans should be discussed with a consultant before their admission for elective surgery. Table 4.1 summarises the Association of Anaesthetists of Great Britain and Ireland indications for the most frequently used tests.

SCORING SYSTEMS

The following scoring systems allow you to grade the risk to the patient and are used to discuss cases with colleagues.

BOX 4.2 The Association of Anaesthesiologists (ASA) grading of physical status is the simplest and most commonly used before surgery[4]

- ASA 1: No systemic disease
- ASA 2: Mild systemic disease
- ASA 3: Severe systemic disease that occasionally threatens life
- ASA 4: Severe systemic disease that constantly threatens life
- ASA 5: Moribund patient who will not survive without surgery
- ASA 6: Brain-dead patient whose organs are being removed for donation

BOX 4.3 The National Institute for Health and Clinical Excellence grading of surgical severity[1]

- Grade 1: Excision skin lesion, breast biopsy
- Grade 2: Inguinal hernia repair, tonsillectomy, knee arthroscopy
- Grade 3: Hysterectomy, thyroidectomy, lumber discectomy
- Grade 4: Total joint replacement, bowel or lung resection

Key points
- Your preoperative visit is your chance to meet your patient, develop a rapport and allay his or her fears.
- Take a history and examination that allows you to gain a summary of the patient's past medical history.
- Decide how these and the surgery will affect your anaesthetic.
- What is the risk to the patient and what will his or her post-operative course be like?
- Decide on post-operative analgesia.
- Only order investigations that will inform your practice. Don't delay surgery for unnecessary tests.

REFERENCES

1. National Institute for Health and Clinical Excellence. *Preoperative Tests: the use of routine preoperative tests for elective surgery; NICE guideline 3*. London: NIHCE; 2003. www.nice.org.uk/guidance/CG3
2. Association of Anaesthetists of Great Britain and Ireland. *Pre-operative Assessment and Patient Preparation: the role of the anaesthetist 2*. London: AAGBI; 2010.
3. Smith TB, Stonell C, Purkayastha S, *et al*. Cardiopulmonary exercise testing as a risk assessment method in non cardio-pulmonary surgery: a systematic review. *Anaesthesia*. 2009; **64**(8): 883–93.
4. www.asahq.org/Home/For-Members/Clinical-Information/ASA-Physical-Status-Classification-System

CHAPTER 5

Intra-operative patient monitoring

JESS BRIGGS AND SHONDIPON LAHA

Monitoring is fundamental to the safe conduct of anaesthesia. If used and interpreted correctly, monitoring devices aid in the early detection of patient deterioration and human error, reducing the risks associated with anaesthesia. Monitoring devices are not a substitute for continued clinical assessment but should be used to alert the anaesthetist to rapidly changing situations.

In this chapter we will cover the basics of essential monitoring and outline some of the more advanced forms of monitoring you may see used.

ASSOCIATION OF ANAESTHETISTS OF GREAT BRITAIN AND IRELAND GUIDELINES FOR MINIMAL MONITORING

The Association of Anaesthetists of Great Britain and Ireland has defined a list of minimum standards of monitoring (*see* Box 5.1), which must be adhered to for every anaesthetic you perform.[1] This includes cases under general or regional anaesthesia, procedures under sedation, local anaesthesia and any transfers you may undertake with a patient. In addition, the following points must also be adhered to.

- Monitors must be checked before use and set suitable audible alarm limits for your patient.
- Core monitoring must be attached prior to induction of anaesthesia. This is not always possible with an uncooperative child. However, there are few, if any, cases where an oxygen saturation probe cannot be attached to even the most fractious child.
- Core data (O_2 saturations, heart rate, blood pressure) must be recorded on the anaesthetic chart every 5 minutes as a minimum standard.

GENERAL GUIDANCE FOR THE USE OF MONITORS

There will be times when the monitors display erroneous values or when the values given do not correlate with the clinical information. Believe your patient and make a rapid assessment of his or her clinical state. Review both the patient and monitors and if in doubt call for help early.

In every hospital monitoring devices differ – it is sensible to ask a senior colleague or friendly operating department practitioner to go through the monitors with you on day one. You will be expected to know:

- how each component (blood pressure cuff, arterial transducer, and so forth) attaches to the monitor and how to check these components and where spares are kept
- how to 'zero' transducers for invasive monitoring, initiate a non-invasive blood pressure reading and set the cuff to cycle at 3- to 5-minute intervals
- how to change alarm settings, apply a temporary silence and how to review a trend screen.

BOX 5.1 Association of Anaesthetists of Great Britain and Ireland minimum monitoring standards[1]

- *The most important monitor is you* – the presence of a suitably trained anaesthetist throughout is mandatory. Clinical assessment should include:
  - mucosal / skin colour, pupil size, response to surgical stimuli
  - movements of the chest wall and reservoir bag (if spontaneously breathing)
  - palpation of the pulse, auscultation of breath sounds
  - monitoring of urine output and blood loss may be required.
- *For induction and maintenance:*
  - core monitoring – pulse oximeter, blood pressure (non-invasive or invasive), electrocardiogram (ECG)
  - inspired oxygen analyser and capnography
  - inspired and expired concentrations of volatile gases (if used)
  - airway pressure monitor
  - the availability of a nerve stimulator and temperature monitor
  - additional monitoring may be required e.g. cardiac output, intracranial pressure monitors.
- *For recovery:*
  - pulse oximeter and blood pressure monitoring
  - the availability of capnography, ECG, nerve stimulator and temperature monitoring.
- *For procedures under sedation or regional or local anaesthesia:*
  - pulse oximeter, blood pressure and ECG.
- *For transfer:*
  - short transfers to a nearby recovery area may be undertaken without monitoring
  - longer transfers require core monitoring and capnography – the addition of airway pressure monitors and inspired oxygen analysers will depend whether a portable ventilator is used or the patient is manually ventilated with a Water's circuit.

PULSE OXIMETRY

What is it?

The humble 'sats probe' allows a non-invasive, beat-to-beat measurement of the oxygen saturation of haemoglobin and the heart rate and gives evidence of the presence of a cardiac output.

In essence this monitor tells you how pink (oxygenated haemoglobin) or blue (relative increase in deoxygenated haemoglobin) your patient is. It is one of the most important monitors in anaesthesia.

How does it work?

The physical principle is based on the differing absorption spectra of oxygenated haemoglobin (HbO_2) compared with deoxygenated haemoglobin (Hb). The probe uses LEDs to emit pulses of red (wavelength, 660 nm) and infrared (wavelength, 940 nm) light, which are absorbed by the Hb and HbO_2 and the tissues. A photocell detects the remaining light on the opposite side of the digit.

The effects of tissue thickness, ambient light, skin pigmentation and venous blood are accounted for and the resulting percentage is based on the ratio of HbO_2:Hb in the pulsatile component of blood. HbO_2 absorbs very little red light and so the red colour predominates, giving a high value for oxygen saturation (and a pink patient!). The opposite applies for deoxygenated haemoglobin (*see* Figure 5.1).

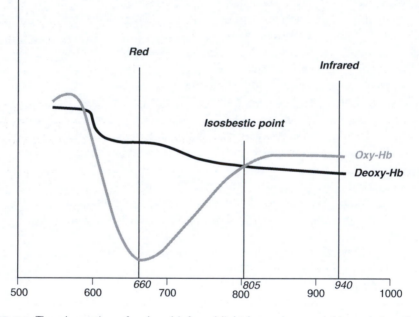

FIGURE 5.1 The absorption of red and infrared light by oxyhaemoglobin and deoxyhaemoglobin, with the isobestic point

Common errors

The machine's algorithms were calibrated against human volunteers, hence values below 80% are unreliable. A poor signal can be caused by a reduction in peripheral perfusion or cardiac output, an increase in venous congestion, an incorrectly positioned probe or movements such as shivering. Check your patient, other monitors and then the probe's position.

Falsely high readings can be caused by carboxyhaemoglobin. Falsely low readings are caused by methaemoglobin, bilirubin, methylene blue dye (used in breast surgery) and nail polish. Detection of cyanosis requires a minimum haemoglobin of 5 g/dL.

In severe anaemia the oxygen saturations may be adequate although your patient is severely hypoxic. In this circumstance an arterial line and direct arterial blood sampling is essential.

Tips for use

The probe is better positioned on the opposite limb to the blood pressure cuff, as your reading will temporarily disappear when the cuff inflates and blood flow is lost distally. Different positions (e.g. fingers or toes) can often improve the signal. An ear probe is useful with a cold shutdown patient and can be placed on ears, lips and nostrils.

For a wriggling child (or agitated granny) certain probes that can be taped to a finger or toe are very useful. Ensure the probe is positioned somewhere that will still be accessible once the patient is draped – there is nothing worse than having to rummage near the nether regions of a surgeon when the probe falls off during surgery.

Be wary as probes can cause both burns and pressure sores during prolonged use.

ELECTROCARDIOGRAM

What is it?

An electrocardiogram (ECG) is a graphical representation of the electrical component of the cardiac cycle giving information on the heart rate, rhythm, conduction and ischaemic changes.

How does it work?

The vector sum of the myocardial cell action potentials are conducted via electrodes and transmitted to the monitor for graphical display by an oscilloscope. This results in a simplified pattern of cardiac electrical activity along axes set up by the sticky electrodes.

'Electrode' refers to the pad that allows electrical conduction, whereas 'lead' refers to the potential difference between two electrodes. A typical '3-lead ECG' can display leads I, II and III from a typical 12-lead ECG. Lead II is most commonly used for continuous display to give the best detection of arrhythmias and P waves.

The leads are placed:

- **R**ed on **R**ight arm/shoulder
- ye**L**low on **L**eft arm
- green/black on left flank/leg.

Placing the 3-lead ECG in the 'CM5' position (red over manubrium; yellow in fifth intercostal space anterior axillary line; green/black over left clavicle) and selecting 'lead I' allows you to monitor V5. This allows better detection of left ventricular ischaemia (in 80%). A 5-lead ECG is also available, which provides more accurate detection of ischaemia.

Common errors

Interference is common from movement artefact, diathermy and occasionally other electrical equipment. These can all give inaccurate visual and numerical displays.

Tips for use

Electrodes commonly fall off (usually the green lead) and the ECG trace will disappear so ensure good placement pre-operatively. You may have to clean or shave the skin and apply adhesive tape over the electrode to ensure good contact. You can vary the lead viewed, electrode position and size of waveform to get the best ECG trace for that patient.

If interference is affecting the display check your patient's pulse to assess for actual arrhythmias (the pulse oximeter will also display heart rate). The presence of CO_2 and arterial line traces also provide reassurance of a cardiac output. Some manufacturers provide electronic filters that reduce the effects of diathermy on the ECG display. You can always ask the surgeon to temporarily stop diathermy to check the rhythm.

INDIRECT BLOOD PRESSURE MONITORING
What is it?
A cuff is used to electronically or manually (using Kortikoff sounds) measure arterial blood pressure.

How does it work?
It is most commonly an automatic pressurised cuff that allows both inflation and detection of arterial wall movements. They were originally designed to measure mean arterial pressure (MAP); however, newer devices also measure systolic pressure and the diastolic is calculated.

Common errors
Shivering or movement artefact (patient or surgeon) can cause failure to detect the pulse. Too large a cuff size under-reads, too narrow over-reads. Automatic blood pressure machines over-read when blood pressure is high and under-read when blood pressure is low. The MAP will remain the most accurate value.

Tips for use
If there is doubt over the accuracy of the blood pressure reading, assess the pulse volume clinically. Change the cuff and its location. Be prepared to insert an invasive arterial line.

INVASIVE ARTERIAL BLOOD PRESSURE MONITOR
What is it?
A small (20 or 22 G) cannula that is placed in an artery (usually the radial, although ulnar, brachial, femoral and dorsalis pedis can be used) to directly measure the arterial pressure. Information on the cardiac output, stroke volume, contractility, afterload and hypovolaemia can be assessed as well as allowing direct arterial blood sampling (*see* Figure 5.2).

How does it work?
The cannula is attached to a transducer via a pressurised, fluid-filled length of tubing through which the arterial waveform is conducted. The transducer converts mechanical pressure signals to electrical ones that are amplified by the monitor and displayed as waveforms.

The accuracy of the system is based upon good transmission of the pressure wave to the transducer, which relies on a correctly placed cannula and equipment. This

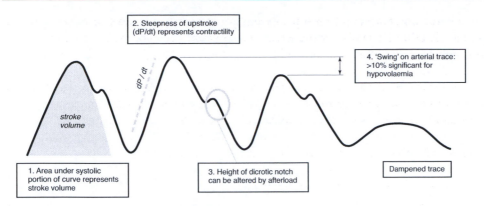

2. Steepness of upstroke (dP/dt) represents contractility

4. 'Swing' on arterial trace: >10% significant for hypovolaemia

dP/dt

stroke volume

1. Area under systolic portion of curve represents stroke volume

3. Height of dicrotic notch can be altered by afterload

Dampened trace

FIGURE 5.2 The arterial pressure waveform, showing inferred measures of stroke volume, contractility, afterload and hypovolaemia – the last waveform is damped

includes specific non-compressible tubing filled with fluid (0.9% or heparinised saline) from a pressurised bag (to 300 mmHg). The fluid line should be 'opened' which allows 3–4 mL/hour to run into the arterial cannula to prevent clots forming. The transducer needs to be level with the patient's heart and 'zeroed' to atmospheric pressure before use.

Common errors

Kinking of the cannula at the skin – ensure the cannula is well sutured and taped in place and that the hand is supported in an optimal position. Clots, bubbles or kinks can give rise to a 'damped' trace (low voltage, small trace). Too long or too flexible tubing causes the system to over-resonate with the mechanical vibrations giving a tall fluctuating trace. While the MAP stays the same, for a given MAP the systolic is higher and the diastolic is lower.

Tips for use

Ensure that the arterial line set has a red stripe along the tubing and red three-way taps – this is to prevent you injecting drugs into the artery.

Ask someone to show you how to:
- set up the line
- zero the transducer
- take blood samples from the three-way tap
- flush the line
- correctly arrange the three-way tap (this is a matter of safety – it can be all too easy to cause an 'anaesthetic haemorrhage' from an incorrectly positioned three-way tap remaining open in the artery).

Attaching the transducer to the patient at the level of the heart prevents you having to move the transducer each time the table is moved.

If the waveform becomes damped:
- flush the line
- try aspirating blood and flushing via the three-way tap with a syringe of saline
- re-zero to atmospheric pressure

- inspect the cannula for kinks, clots and air (these must be aspirated carefully to prevent them from entering the circulation)
- reposition the limb.

A huge amount of information can be gained from this relatively simple monitor – if your patient is sick (especially cardiac patients), obese or requires major surgery or frequent arterial blood gases, then insert an arterial line.

CAPNOGRAPHY

What is it?

A graphical representation of end-tidal expired carbon dioxide (etCO$_2$) against time. The presence of a continued CO$_2$ trace confirms tracheal intubation and shows the presence of a cardiac output. The shape of the trace gives additional information (*see* Figure 5.3).

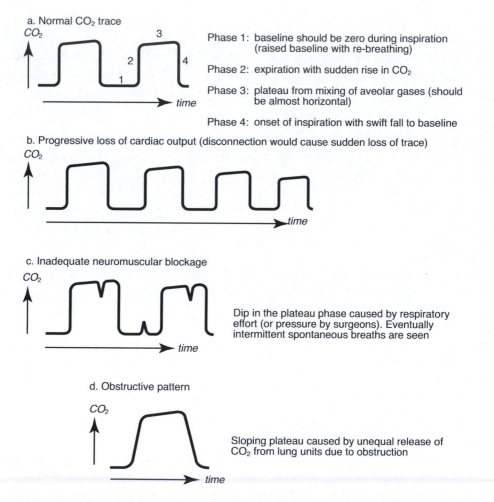

a. Normal CO$_2$ trace

Phase 1: baseline should be zero during inspiration (raised baseline with re-breathing)

Phase 2: expiration with sudden rise in CO$_2$

Phase 3: plateau from mixing of aveolar gases (should be almost horizontal)

Phase 4: onset of inspiration with swift fall to baseline

b. Progressive loss of cardiac output (disconnection would cause sudden loss of trace)

c. Inadequate neuromuscular blockage

Dip in the plateau phase caused by respiratory effort (or pressure by surgeons). Eventually intermittent spontaneous breaths are seen

d. Obstructive pattern

Sloping plateau caused by unequal release of CO$_2$ from lung units due to obstruction

FIGURE 5.3 (a) A normal capnograph trace showing the four phases; (b) a decreasing amplitude indicates a progressive loss of cardiac output; (c) dips in phase III indicate the start of spontaneous respiration after neuromuscular blockade; (d) the obstructive pattern

How does it work?

Measurement is usually via an infrared detector, which can be attached directly to the breathing circuit (heavy and cumbersome but with fewer delays) or suctioned through a small side arm to a detection chamber on the monitor (most common type but with slightly increased delay).

Dead space gas (the proportion exposed only to conducting airways and therefore containing no CO_2) mixes with alveolar gas to form the expired tidal volume and CO_2 trace. The $etCO_2$ is therefore 0.3–0.7 kPa lower than the alveolar (and arterial) pCO_2 in healthy subjects. Where there is poor diffusion of CO_2 across alveolar membranes or poor ventilation, the arterial pCO_2 may be much higher than the $etCO_2$.

Common errors

Moisture in the system can cause erroneous readings. Kinking or standing on the sampling tubing and disconnection or leaks in the breathing circuit or sampling line can cause loss of trace.

Tips for use

Capnography is one of the most important monitors in anaesthesia. Do not be tempted to intubate or transfer a patient without it. As with all monitors, if there is a problem with the CO_2 trace, check your patient first and then check the monitor.

OXYGEN ANALYSER

What is it?

An O_2 analyser is an analyser to confirm the concentration of oxygen being delivered to the patient. It acts as a final safety check (cases have occurred where a gas other than oxygen has been connected to the gas supply and thus a hypoxic mixture delivered to the patient). It should sample inspiratory gases as close to the patient as possible. It displays the oxygen concentration (partial pressure) as a percentage of the total gas flow.

How does it work?

It is normally incorporated inside the newer anaesthetic machines. There are several types of analysers using differing principles (polargraphic, fuel cell, paramagnetic).

Common errors

Ask an operating department practitioner to show you the analysers used on your anaesthetic machines and how to check them. Normally these are calibrated in air and then 100% O_2. Water vapour can be problematic and a water trap is present – this needs checking to ensure it is not overfull.

ANALYSERS FOR ANAESTHETIC VAPOURS

What is it?

It is vital that the anaesthetic vapours delivered to the patient are measured in both the patient's inspired and the patient's expired concentrations. While the inspired concentration relates to the amount of vapour delivered to the patient (dependent on the concentration from the vaporiser, fresh gas flow in the circuit and breathing system in use), the expired concentration is a better reflection of blood and therefore brain concentrations of the agent.

How does it work?

Gases sampled from the breathing system are analysed using infrared detectors in a chamber with the gases then returned to the system, giving breath-by-breath analysis. The gas is taken from the same sample line as the CO_2 and O_2.

Common errors

The problems are similar to CO_2 sample lines. Water vapour is not a problem with infrared detectors; however, nebulised salbutamol in the breathing system may be identified as halothane by certain anaesthetic machines (e.g. Dräger Primus).

TEMPERATURE MONITORING

This should be used in all but routine short cases. It can be intermittent via tympanic membrane thermometers (core temperature) during short cases or with continuous monitors.

Continuous monitoring can be via a nasopharyngeal probe, although this is only accurate in ventilated patients where airflow does not occur over the probe tip. Core body temperature can be measured via oesophageal probes (risk of perforation) or via specialised urinary catheters and intracranial monitoring. Rectal temperature significantly lags behind core temperature.

CARDIAC OUTPUT MONITORS

There are many cardiac output monitors in use and only brief details will be given here. Most departments will have one type of cardiac output monitor available for use. You would be wise to ask for a demonstration and use it alongside the consultant during appropriate cases.

All cardiac output monitors have limitations and all make assumptions in order to derive the information – which monitor you use will depend on familiarity and availability. The accuracy is increased when the trends and responses to clinical interventions (e.g. fluid challenges or use of inotropes) are used as opposed to one-off readings. Clinical markers (skin perfusion, urine output, and lactate) should always be used in conjunction with derived data.

In order to use cardiac output monitors it is useful to first review your cardiac physiology.

- Cardiac output = stroke volume × heart rate.
- Blood pressure = cardiac output × systemic vascular resistance.
- Stroke volume is dependent on preload (ventricular filling), contractility and afterload (ventricular outflow resistance including systemic vascular resistance).
- Oxygen delivery = cardiac output × arterial O_2 content.
- Indexes (e.g. cardiac index) are the value in question divided by the body surface area (m^2).

OESOPHAGEAL DOPPLER MONITOR

A flexible probe is positioned in the distal-oesophagus, which lies adjacent to the descending aorta. The tip contains a Doppler transducer. Emitted ultrasound waves bounce off red blood cells descending in the aorta. The velocity of these cells can be determined and thus stroke volume and cardiac output obtained.

Accurate positioning can be difficult – make small adjustments and listen for the optimal Doppler sound. If the monitor is to be used throughout theatre, taping the probe to the tracheal tube may help keep it in place. There is a risk of oesophageal perforation.

VIGILEO, LiDCO

Although different, both Vigileo and LiDCO monitors mathematically derive cardiac output from the arterial trace and both require attachments or separate transducer kits on the arterial line. The LiDCO uses lithium to calibrate the monitor, although there is now an uncalibrated version (LiDCO Plus) which is more suitable for theatre use.

PULMONARY ARTERY (SWAN–GANZ) CATHETER

The pulmonary artery (Swan–Ganz) catheter was the 'gold standard' for monitoring cardiac output, although it is infrequently used now because of the risks from insertion and dilation of the pulmonary balloon component. It involved inserting a catheter via the internal jugular, through the right atrium and then the ventricle before inflating a balloon that allowed it to wedge in the pulmonary vasculature. This resulted in a theoretical column of fluid from the tip to the left atrium highlighting left heart-filling pressures. The cardiac output could be derived by injecting a known volume of cold fluid at a certain temperature into the right atrium and measuring the corresponding thermal dip at the tip of the catheter with a thermistor. The thermodilution curve that is generated can then be used to derive the cardiac output.

OTHER MONITORS

Bispectral index monitoring assesses the electrical activity in the brain and the depth of anaesthesia – used mainly to avoid patient awareness.

Neuromuscular monitoring is used in the presence of paralysing drugs (*see* Chapter 16).

Key points

- You are the most important monitor. You must continually make clinical assessments of your patient, especially if the monitor is misreading.
- ECG, non-invasive blood pressure, oxygen saturations and capnography are essential. Other more complicated monitors may be used as required.
- Make sure that you learn the potential errors of each measurement system and how to troubleshoot them.

REFERENCE

1. Association of Anaesthetists of Great Britain and Ireland. *Standards of Monitoring During Anaesthesia and Recovery.* 4th ed. London: AAGBI; 2007.

CHAPTER 6

The anaesthetic machine

ANNA CROSBY AND SHONDIPON LAHA

BACKGROUND

The first purpose-built anaesthetic machine was developed in 1917 by the British anaesthetist Henry Boyle (1875–1941). Even with all the advances in the field of anaesthesia since then modern machines retain the same essential components as the original Boyle model. Even the knobs are still based on left-handed use, as Boyle was himself left-handed.

One of the simplest ways to remember these components is to think of the machines in terms of the route the gases take as they travel from the pipelines or cylinders through the system to the common gas outlet.

GAS SUPPLY (PIPELINE OR CYLINDERS)

- Pressure gauges
- Pressure regulators and valves
- Rotameters/flowmeters
- Vaporisers
- Common gas outlet

The anaesthetic machine is a fundamental piece of equipment and it is a basic requirement that all anaesthetists understand how it works and how to check it. Anaesthetic machines should be checked at the start of every operating session, with additional checks being carried out for each new patient or in the event of any equipment changes (e.g. vaporiser change).

Although some machine checks may be carried out by an anaesthetic assistant or operating department practitioner, it is ultimately the responsibility of the anaesthetist to make sure everything is in order and you should always make sure that you have carried out the checks yourself as well and recorded the information on your anaesthetic chart.

Pipeline gas

Piped medical gases and vacuum are delivered throughout the hospital from central supply points such as liquid oxygen tanks or cylinder banks at an average pressure of

400 kPa within the pipes. Each of the four gas outlets in theatres is not only named but also colour-coded:

- oxygen (O_2) – white
- nitrous oxide (N_2O) – blue
- compressed air – black
- suctioning – yellow.

They are fitted with a unique socket, the 'Schrader' valve, designed to accept only corresponding, colour-coded gas hoses from the anaesthetic machine.

A second safety feature is the non-interchangeable screw-thread located at the junction between the gas hose and the anaesthetic machine. This is again gas specific and should be permanently fixed.

These inbuilt safety mechanisms prevent any crossover between gas flows from the outlets through the piping and into the anaesthetic machine, which can cause delivery of a hypoxic gas mixture.

Cylinder gas

In the event of pipeline failure there is reserve O_2 and N_2O stored in the size E cylinders at the back of the anaesthetic machine.

The exact pressure within the cylinders is dependent upon the gas contained within it. A full O_2 cylinder at room temperature stores O_2 in the gas state at 13,700 kPa, this pressure decreases in a linear manner as the cylinder empties. N_2O at room temperature on the other hand exists in the liquid/vapour state and, when full, is pressurised to 4400 kPa.

Unlike O_2, as the N_2O cylinder empties the contents gradually shift from the liquid to the vapour state. This maintains a constant pressure in the cylinder until all the contents exist in the vapour state; further emptying beyond this point will cause the pressure to fall – this occurs when the cylinder is about a quarter full.

Cylinders are also colour-coded for safety. Therefore, at the back of your anaesthetic machine you should see O_2, black body and white shoulders, and N_2O, blue body and blue shoulders.

On the neck of the cylinder is a screw thread into which a brass valve is fitted. These are opened using a key, or in the case of newer cylinders, a handle incorporated into the valve. The valve provides an important safety mechanism known as the pin index system. Each valve has two drilled holes; these are specifically positioned and identify the gas contained within the cylinder. They are designed to match a corresponding arrangement of pins located on the cylinder ports ('yokes') of the anaesthetic machine. If an attempt is made to fit the wrong cylinder to the yoke, the exit port of the cylinder will not seal against the washer (a specially designed Bodok seal) on the yoke, leaving a leak between the cylinder and the machine.

PRESSURE GAUGES

It is important to check the pressures from both sources as they enter. 'Bourdon' pressure gauges measuring the pressure in the gases delivered from both the pipelines and the cylinders can be found mounted on the front of the anaesthetic machine. In the event of damage to the tube, gas vents out through the back of the gauge rather than through the reinforced glass at the front.

As with the pipelines and cylinders, the pressure gauges are colour-coded to help ensure accurate readings, as the gauges are calibrated to specific gases. However, it is important that the gauge is measuring not only the correct gas but also the correct source (i.e. cylinder or pipeline), as the higher cylinder pressures would damage a gauge designed for only pipeline pressures.

PRESSURE-REDUCING VALVES

The purpose of the pressure-reducing valves is to convert the high and variable pressures from the cylinders into a constant pressure just below that of pipeline pressure (i.e. 400 kPa). This allows delivery of constant flows from the cylinders and protects the rest of the anaesthetic machine from high-pressure damage.

Pressure-reducing valves consist of two chambers separated by a valve attached to a diaphragm. Cylinder gas enters the first chamber and passes through the valve to the second chamber along a pressure gradient. As the pressure in the second chamber rises, the volume of the chamber moves the diaphragm. This causes the attached valve to close, preventing further gas flow into the second chamber. As the pressure falls, the sprung diaphragm returns to its original position, allowing the valve to re-open and the process to begin again.

ONE-WAY VALVES

Gases are prevented from back-flowing through the pressure-reducing valves and leaving the system by means of one-way valves.

RELIEF VALVES

In the event of failure of the pressure-reducing valves, there are relief valves situated downstream that allow gas to escape once the pressure rises above a fixed point (commonly 700 kPa).

SECOND-STAGE REGULATORS AND FLOW RESTRICTORS

Pipeline pressures can also be subject to surges. These can be controlled with either pressure regulators, as described earlier, or flow restrictors, which are simply a constriction between the pipeline supply and the anaesthetic machine.

FLOW CONTROL (NEEDLE) VALVES

Flow control or 'needle' valves allow manual adjustment of the flow through rotameters. There is one brass valve situated at the base of each pair of rotameter tubes that may be adjusted by means of a labelled, colour-coded knob. When the knob is turned anticlockwise the screw thread moves the end of the needle outwards, which opens up the valve allowing increased flow through the rotameter.

The knob controlling the O_2 valve is larger than for other gases, with grooves cut into the side. This is a safety feature that allows quick identification of the O_2 even in the dark! Another means of quick identification is the UK convention that always places the O_2 knob to the left of other gases.

ROTAMETERS

Rotameters or flowmeters are found grouped in a unit on the front of traditional anaesthetic machines; newer machines tend to have digital readings of gas flows. The purpose of the rotameters is to measure the flow rate of gases passing through them. The back panel of the rotameter unit is often illuminated. Each rotameter consists of a tapered glass or transparent plastic tube in which a rotating bobbin (most common) or ball floats giving a measure of the flow rate. The higher the gas flow the further the bobbin or ball will move up the tube. At the top of each tube there is a wire stop to prevent the bobbin or ball moving partially or totally out of view and therefore preventing an accurate reading. When adjusting the flow on the rotameters, readings should be taken from the top if using a bobbin or from the centre if using a ball. Although both the tubes and bobbins are designed to prevent sticking, it is important to check that the bobbin is rotating and is able to move freely, allowing accurate readings to be made; for this purpose each bobbin is marked with a dot.

Rotameters are non-interchangeable, being calibrated at room temperature and atmospheric pressure to a specific gas. If you look at a rotameter tube you can see that the interval between each calibration point is not equal, the graduations get closer together higher up the tube because of its tapered nature.

Each of the anaesthetic gases has two rotameter tubes that are controlled by a single flow control needle valve. The first tube measures flows up to 1 L/minute, allowing accurate adjustment at very low flows, while the second measures flows up to 15 L/minute.

Although, as explained earlier, UK convention places the O_2 rotameter and knob to the left of the other gases; O_2 is actually the last gas to join the back bar at the top right-hand side of the rotameter unit. This is to preserve the O_2 supply in the event of damage to any of the other rotameters. The interactive O_2 and N_2O controls prevent delivery of a hypoxic gas mixture by ensuring that when N_2O levels are above a certain point there will be a proportional rise in the O_2 flow.

VAPORISERS

The gases then pass along the back bar to the vaporisers, where controlled quantities of volatile anaesthetic agents are passed into the fresh gas flow. In the UK the more advanced plenum vaporisers, which allow more controlled delivery of vapours, tend to be used; however, simpler draw over systems also exist.

Vaporisers are found on the back bar of the anaesthetic machine seated on two port valves. At the junction between the vaporiser and each valve are O-ring washers that prevent leaks. Only when the vaporiser is locked in position and turned on can the fresh gas flow enter.

Often there will be more than one vaporiser seated on the back bar. As each vaporiser is designed to carry a single volatile agent, an interlocking 'Selectatec' system prevents transfer of upstream agents to the downstream vaporiser and simultaneous delivery of two agents. Another feature to prevent cross-contamination of vaporisers is the uniquely shaped filling port that only fits the compatible, colour-coded volatile agent bottle. This safety filling system also ensures that the vaporisers cannot overflow and reduces incidence of spillage.

COMMON GAS OUTLET

The final fresh gas flow/vapour mix exits the anaesthetic machine via the common gas outlet; it is here that the O_2 analyser is situated (before the gas mixture enters the patient). The pressure of the gas is now at approximately atmospheric pressure, with most of the drop from the pipeline pressures having occurred across the rotameters.

OTHER IMPORTANT FEATURES

Non-return pressure safety relief valve

In addition to the valves described earlier, a further non-return pressure safety relief valve is situated downstream of the vaporisers. It may be either on the back bar or near the common gas outlet. Like the valves already described, its purpose is to protect the components of the anaesthetic machine in the event of excess pressure. In this case, back pressure due to obstruction at or near the common gas outlet. The valve is released when pressures exceed 35 kPa.

Emergency O_2 flush

The emergency O_2 flush delivers pure O_2 to the common gas outlet. This is activated by a white, labelled button situated near the outlet.

As the emergency O_2 flush allows O_2 from the pipelines and cylinders to bypass the rotameters and vaporisers the O_2 is delivered at a pressure of about 400 kPa and a flow rate of 35–75 L/minute. These higher pressures and flow rates can put patients at increased risk of barotrauma. It is also important to note that as the O_2 is not passing through the vaporiser it is free from any anaesthetic agent and therefore if used it will dilute any inhalational agents, increasing the potential for patient awareness.

O_2 supply failure alarm

The O_2 supply failure alarm is an audible alarm that creates a special sound unique to all the other 'beeps' and alert sounds produced by the anaesthetic machine. It is designed to activate when the O_2 pressure falls and it is able to alert even in the presence of a total power failure, being independent of both battery and mains supplies.

CHECKING THE ANAESTHETIC MACHINE

The Association of Anaesthetists of Great Britain and Ireland provide a checklist for anaesthetic machines.[1] A laminated copy of this list should be attached to the anaesthetic machines and is a useful reminder of what you should be checking (*see* Appendix 2).

The following checks should be made prior to each operating session. In addition, checks 2, 6 and 9 (Monitoring, Breathing System and Ancillary Equipment) should be made prior to each new patient during a session.

1. **Check that the anaesthetic machine is connected to the electricity supply (if appropriate) and switched on. Note:** some anaesthetic workstations may enter an integral self-test programme when switched on; those functions tested by such a programme need not be retested.
   - Take note of any information or labelling on the anaesthetic machine referring to the current status of the machine. Particular attention should be paid to recent servicing. Servicing labels should be fixed in the service logbook.
2. **Check that all monitoring devices, in particular the O_2 analyser, pulse oximeter and capnograph, are functioning and have appropriate alarm limits.**
   - Check that gas sampling lines are properly attached and free of obstructions.

- Check that an appropriate frequency of recording non-invasive blood pressure is selected.
- (Some monitors need to be in stand-by mode to avoid unnecessary alarms before being connected to the patient).

3. **Check with a 'tug test' that each pipeline is correctly inserted into the appropriate gas supply terminal. Note:** carbon dioxide cylinders should not be present on the anaesthetic machine unless requested by the anaesthetist. A blanking plug should be fitted to any empty cylinder yoke.
   - Check that the anaesthetic machine is connected to a supply of O_2 and that an adequate supply of O_2 is available from a reserve O_2 cylinder.
   - Check that adequate supplies of other gases (N_2O, air) are available and connected as appropriate.
   - Check that all pipeline pressure gauges in use on the anaesthetic machine indicate 400–500 kPa.

4. **Check the operation of flowmeters (where fitted).**
   - Check that each flow valve operates smoothly and that the bobbin moves freely throughout its range.
   - Check the anti-hypoxia device is working correctly.
   - Check the operation of the emergency O_2 bypass control.

5. **Check the vaporiser(s).**
   - Check that each vaporiser is adequately, but not over, filled.
   - Check that each vaporiser is correctly seated on the back bar and not tilted.
   - Check the vaporiser for leaks (with vaporiser on and off) by temporarily occluding the common gas outlet.
   - Turn the vaporiser(s) off when checks are completed.
   - Repeat the leak test immediately after changing any vaporiser.

6. **Check the breathing system to be employed. Note:** a new single use bacterial/viral filter and angle-piece/catheter mount must be used for each patient. Packaging should not be removed until point of use.
   - Inspect the system for correct configuration. All connections should be secured by 'push and twist'.
   - Perform a pressure leak test on the breathing system by occluding the patient-end and compressing the reservoir bag. Bain-type co-axial systems should have the inner tube compressed for the leak test.
   - Check the correct operation of all valves, including unidirectional valves within a circle, and all exhaust valves.
   - Check for patency and flow of gas through the whole breathing system including the filter and anglepiece/catheter mount.

7. **Check that the ventilator is configured appropriately for its intended use.**
   - Check that the ventilator tubing is correctly configured and securely attached.
   - Set the controls for use and ensure that an adequate pressure is generated during the inspiratory phase.
   - Check the pressure relief valve functions.
   - Check that the disconnect alarms function correctly.
   - Ensure that an alternative means to ventilate the patient's lungs is available. (see 10. below)

8. **Check that the anaesthetic gas scavenging system is switched on and is functioning correctly.**
   - Check that the tubing is attached to the appropriate exhaust port of the breathing system, ventilator or workstation.
9. **Check that all ancillary equipment that may be needed is present and working.**
   - This includes laryngoscopes, intubation aids, intubation forceps, bougies etc. and appropriately sized face masks, airways, tracheal tubes and connectors, which must be checked for patency.
   - Check that the suction apparatus is functioning and that all connectors are secure.
   - Check that the patient trolley, bed or operating table can be rapidly tilted head down.
10. **Check that an alternative means to ventilate the patient is immediately available (e.g. self-inflating bag and O_2 cylinder).**
    - Check that the self-inflating bag and cylinder of O_2 are functioning correctly and the cylinder contains an adequate supply of O_2.
11. **Recording**
    - Sign and date the logbook kept with the anaesthetic machine to confirm the machine has been checked.
    - Record on each patient's anaesthetic chart that the anaesthetic machine, breathing system and monitoring equipment have been checked.

To help avoid forgetting any steps it is helpful to develop a routine, dividing the machine into sections and checking each section by turn. Once you understand your machine and you know that its working and you know what you will do if it stops working you can start to gain confidence using it.

Key points
- Understanding the anaesthetic machine is a key part of delivering anaesthesia.
- The anaesthetist is responsible for making sure that it is functioning safely.
- Compliance with the Association of Anaesthetists of Great Britain and Ireland guidance is mandatory practice.

REFERENCE

1. Hartle A, Anderson E, Bythell V, *et al.* Association of Anaesthetists of Great Britain and Ireland. Checking anaesthetic equipment 2012. *Anaesthesia.* 2012; **67**(6): 660–8.

CHAPTER 7

Anaesthetic breathing systems

JUSTIN ROBERTS AND LEANNE DARWIN

Defined as a series of components, predominantly a reservoir bag, tubing and an adjustable pressure-limiting (APL) valve that connect the patient's airway to the gas delivery device, breathing systems have been classified in numerous, often unhelpful, ways. Broadly, breathing systems are divided into those that incorporate a system for carbon dioxide (CO_2) absorption and those that do not. Other commonly used classifications are the closed (all expired gas rebreathed), semi-closed (proportion of expired rebreathed) and open systems. An example of an open system would be the dripping of ether or chloroform onto a face mask – this is not used these days and therefore won't be explored further here.

A quick tip on valves: Turn to the Left to Loosen

THE CIRCLE SYSTEM

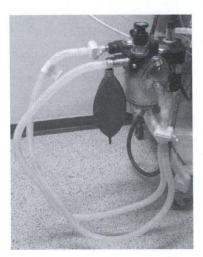

FIGURE 7.1 The circle circuit

The circle system is a fully closed circuit and typically consists of:

- fresh gas entry point
- unidirectional valves (inspiratory and expiratory)
- reservoir bag
- CO_2 absorption device (soda lime)
- APL valve
- Y-piece for connection to the patient.

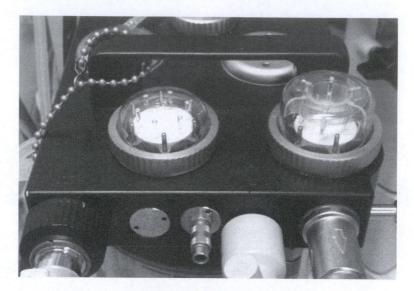

FIGURE 7.2 Unidirectional valves prevent backwards flow in the circle circuit

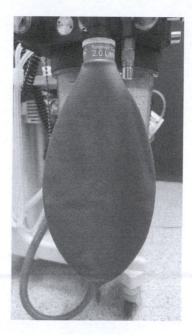

FIGURE 7.3 A reservoir bag

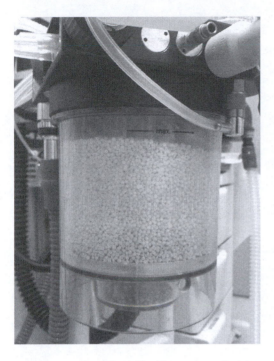

FIGURE 7.4 Soda lime absorbs carbon dioxide from the circle, allowing the gases to be reused

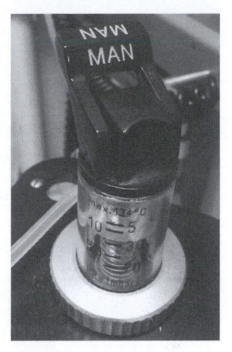

FIGURE 7.5 The adjustable pressure-limiting valve allows the pressure to set in the circuit so that the patient can be manually ventilated

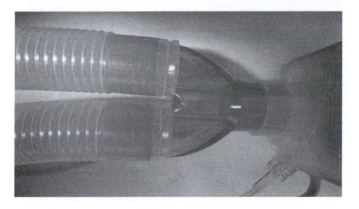

FIGURE 7.6 The Y-piece connects the circuit to the patient

The soda lime in the circle circuit means that the patient can rebreathe the gases in the circuit. Once the dose of volatile gas in the patient has reached a steady state then the fresh gas flow into the circuit can be reduced. Below 1 L/minute is 'low-flow anaesthesia'. This must only be performed with inspired and expired gas monitoring, as the concentrations of oxygen and volatile gas in the fresh gas flow are not the same as in the circuit. It will take you a little time to get experienced enough to use low-flow anaesthesia. It has the potential for hypoxic gas mixtures and patient awareness.

The circle system has a number of advantages, particularly when used with low fresh gas flows:

- economical (considerable financial savings to be made with lower flows – clinical directors love to audit this!)
- humidification (retains humidity from expired gases)
- heat retention (heat from expired gases and heat produced when soda lime absorbs CO_2 help maintain the patient's temperature)
- reduction in atmospheric pollution.

SEMI-CLOSED BREATHING SYSTEMS

These are so called as the patient rebreathes a proportion of the gas he or she expires, but not all of it (as in the circle). In 1954, W. Mapleson, a Cardiff physicist, classified semi-closed breathing systems from A to E, determining their efficiency upon the theoretical fresh gas flow (FGF) required to prevent the rebreathing of CO_2. The Mapleson F system was added at a later date.

Mapleson A

The Mapleson A is also known as a 'Magill's' circuit. It consists of a T-tube connected to the fresh gas flow outlet, a reservoir bag, reservoir tubing, and an APL valve at the patient end of the circuit. The flow required to prevent rebreathing is as follows:

Spontaneous ventilation: FGF = alveolar ventilation or 70 mL/kg/minute
Controlled ventilation: FGF = 150 mL/kg/minute.

Although very efficient for spontaneous breathing patients, it is rather unusual to see this system in use.

The co-axial version (where one of the arms of the T-piece is within the other) is the Lack circuit, where inspiration occurs from the outer reservoir tube and expiration into the inner exhaust tube. Properties are similar to the Magill's circuit, but the APL valve is more conveniently located, at the anaesthetic machine end of the circuit.

Mapleson B

The Mapleson B is very infrequently used and only of interest for exam purposes! The FGF inlet is close to the patient, between the APL valve and the reservoir tubing. Similar physical properties to the Mapleson C, a FGF of twice the minute ventilation for both spontaneous and controlled ventilation.

Mapleson C

Commonly referred to as a Waters' circuit, this system is found throughout hospitals including post-operative recovery areas and emergency department resuscitation areas. It is infrequently used for the induction and maintenance of anaesthesia because of its inefficiency, requiring 1.5–2 times minute ventilation. It is popular for a number of reasons:

- portability
- the proximity of the APL valve and reservoir bag to the patient
- the ability to apply continuous positive airway pressure with partial closure of the APL valve plus or minus a face mask

- it allows assisted ventilation
- the feel of the reservoir bag allows assessment of lung compliance
- it is easily attached to an oxygen cylinder in the event of an anaesthetic machine or mainline gas delivery failure.

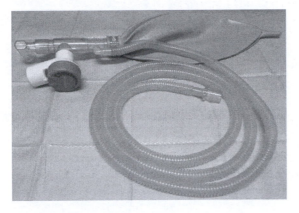

FIGURE 7.7 The Mapleson C circuit

Mapleson D

Commonly seen as the Bain system, which is the co-axial (inspiratory limb is within the expiratory limb) version of the Mapleson D. This is frequently seen within anaesthesia induction rooms but can also be found in emergency department resuscitation areas. Functionally, it is the opposite of the Mapleson A:

Controlled ventilation: FGF = alveolar ventilation or 70 mL/kg/minute
Spontaneous ventilation: FGF = 150 mL/kg/minute.

Any coaxial system carries the disadvantage of potential occult disconnection, resulting in increased dead space.

Mapleson E and F

The Mapleson E or Ayres T-piece is only commonly used during the recovery phase of anaesthesia. There is an inspiratory limb that receives the fresh gas flow and is connected to the patient with a Y-connector. The expiratory limb then acts as a reservoir and some of the exhaled CO_2 is blown out by the fresh gas flow during the patient's expiratory pause. This ensures a fixed FiO_2. Rebreathing of CO_2 is prevented by high FGF, usually two to three times the patient's minute volume.

The Mapleson F or Jackson-Rees system is created by the addition of an open-ended reservoir bag to the expiratory limb of the T-piece. It requires a significant FGF of three times minute ventilation for both spontaneously and mechanically ventilated patients. Its chief use is in paediatric anaesthesia because it allows ventilation with low volumes. Its major disadvantage is the inability to effectively and easily scavenge expelled gases.

There is a modification of the Mapleson F that incorporates an APL valve with a limiting pressure at 30 cmH$_2$O and a closed reservoir bag. This system allows effective scavenging to be added to the APL valve.

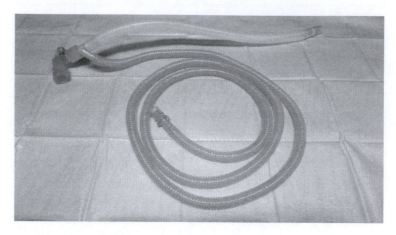

FIGURE 7.8 The Mapleson E circuit

Humphrey ADE

Utilising the advantages of the Mapleson A, D and E systems, the Humphrey ADE is efficient for both spontaneous and mechanical ventilation. However, the Humphrey ADE is infrequently seen in daily clinical practice.

THE SELF-INFLATING BAG

All of the aforementioned systems require a source of fresh gas, whether from a piped wall supply (via an anaesthetic machine or rotameter) or an oxygen cylinder. The self-inflating bag is a vital piece of equipment, particularly when transferring a patient either within or between hospitals, as it allows ventilation with oxygen-enriched air in the event of a ventilator failure. More important, it allows ventilation with air in the event of oxygen supply failure (such as inadequate cylinder supply following lift or ambulance breakdowns!).

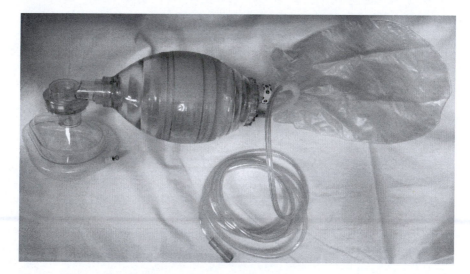

FIGURE 7.9 A self-inflating bag

Key points

- The circle circuit is a closed system. The soda lime removes CO_2 and allows the other gases to be rebreathed.
- The circle is the only circuit that can be used for low-flow anaesthesia.
- Gas monitors must be used during low-flow anaesthesia to prevent hypoxia and patient awareness.
- The Mapleson circuits allow partial rebreathing. Higher fresh gas flows are needed to purge the CO_2 from the circuit.
- Self-inflating bags are essential during transfers, as they are the only circuit that does not require a gas source to drive it.

CHAPTER 8

Ventilation

FIONA WALLACE, CLAIRE ALLEN AND DANIEL COTTLE

INTRODUCTION

There are several reasons to ventilate a patient during anaesthesia.

Airway protection

Anaesthesia depresses protective airway reflexes. Contamination of the lungs may occur as a result of aspiration of stomach contents or from upper airway surgery. You may wish to protect the lungs with an endotracheal tube. Placement usually requires use of a muscle relaxant, rendering the patient apnoeic and in need of ventilation.

Carbon dioxide clearance

Ventilation is the movement of gas in and out of the lungs. Carbon dioxide (CO_2) easily diffuses across membranes and so these movements limit its clearance. Hypoventilation is common under anaesthesia because of anaesthetic agents, opioid analgesia and muscle relaxants. CO_2 clearance is also reduced by ventilation–perfusion mismatch. The efficacy of ventilation is measured by the clearance of CO_2 from the body via the lungs using arterial blood gases or capnography (*see* Chapter 5). Mechanically ventilating a patient may maintain or increase CO_2 clearance.

Oxygenation

Oxygenation depends upon open alveoli taking part in gas exchange. Positive-pressure ventilation can hold open alveoli (recruitment) and ensure oxygenation. It also allows the administration of higher concentrations of oxygen.

During normal respiration, expansion of the chest creates a negative pressure, which draws air into the lungs. Negative pressure can be created externally (e.g. the 'iron lung'). In contrast, most modern ventilators exert a positive pressure, which pushes gas into the lungs, so-called intermittent positive-pressure ventilation.

METHODS OF VENTILATION

Broadly speaking, theatre ventilators will deliver either volume or pressure-controlled ventilation. It is useful to consider the following equations when thinking about ventilation.

Compliance (mL/cmH$_2$O) = volume (mL)/pressure (cmH$_2$O)
Minute volume (mL) = tidal volume (mL) × respiratory rate

VOLUME-CONTROLLED VENTILATION

By setting the tidal volume (Vt) and the respiratory rate you determine the minute volume. This allows you to control the arterial CO$_2$. Volume-controlled ventilation delivers a preset volume at a constant flow rate. Airway pressure therefore increases during inspiration until the selected tidal volume is delivered. The pressure required to deliver the Vt is inversely related to the chest compliance. Reduced compliance will result in high pressures being generated, which can cause barotraumas to the lung (e.g. pneumothorax). This is made worse by any condition that reduces compliance: laparoscopic surgery, obesity, obstructive lung disease or head-down tilt. Appropriate high-pressure limits and alarms must be set; these are normally 30–35 cmH$_2$O.

PRESSURE-CONTROLLED VENTILATION

In contrast, pressure-controlled ventilation delivers a preset pressure, with the flow decelerating throughout inspiration to achieve this. By limiting the pressure you can prevent barotraumas. This time it is the tidal volume that depends on compliance. If the compliance is poor (or the pressure too low) then ventilation will suffer because of a low Vt – subsequently, CO$_2$ rises. If the lung is very compliant (or the pressure is too high) a very high Vt might result – this can then result in volutrauma. You must set the alarm limits for tidal volume and minute ventilation. Pressure-controlled ventilation can improve gas exchange, especially in patients with abnormal lungs because the alveoli are held open for longer.

Laparoscopic procedures are associated with significant changes in compliance due to insufflation of the abdomen and positional changes (e.g. head down for gynaecological laparoscopies). One approach to this situation is to use volume-controlled ventilation with appropriately set alarm limits.

If you decide to use intermittent positive-pressure ventilation with a laryngeal mask airway, pressure-controlled ventilation may be preferable to avoid excessive pressures, which can cause insufflation of the stomach.

PRESSURE SUPPORT VENTILATION

This type of ventilation can be used to support patients making inadequate spontaneous ventilatory effort. The ventilator detects spontaneous inspiratory flow instigated by the patient. It then delivers a pressure-controlled breath at the same time as the patient. It can also be used to overcome the resistance in the breathing circuit or airway. It requires a sophisticated ventilator with microprocessor control.

Positive end-expiratory pressure

Positive end-expiratory pressure (PEEP) is, as the name suggests, a positive pressure maintained at the end of expiration. It prevents alveolar collapse and re-expansion, which can be damaging. By holding open (and recruiting) alveoli it can improve oxygenation. By recruiting lung, PEEP can increase lung compliance and reduce the total pressure required for ventilation. However, PEEP may impede venous return, causing decreased cardiac output and increased intracranial pressure. High levels of

PEEP will increase dead space ventilation. PEEP is rarely needed for healthy lungs or short procedures.

HOW TO SET UP A VENTILATOR

1. Check the ventilator and other associated equipment according to Association of Anaesthetists of Great Britain and Ireland guidelines (*see* Chapter 6).
2. Select an adequate FiO_2.
   › Clearly this will vary from patient to patient.
   › This may be via rotameters or an electronic control.
3. Ensure adequate flow.
   › Circle systems allow for low flow anaesthesia (e.g. less than 1 L/minute). This is economical and good for the environment! (*See* Chapter 7).
   › However, there is a minimum flow required to compensate for uptake by the patient and small leaks in the circuit. The reservoir bag should not completely collapse.
   › If you want to change the concentration of volatile anaesthetic agent or FiO_2, keep in mind that this will take a long time at low flows. If you need to change it quickly, increase flow rates.
4. Set the rate.
   › Normally 10–12 breaths per minute.
5. Select either volume or pressure control.
   › Normal tidal volume is 7–8 mL/kg.
   › For pressure-controlled ventilation the pressure required can vary significantly and should be titrated to tidal volume.
   › Aim to keep the $etCO_2$ in the normal range (4.5–6.0 kPa).
6. Set PEEP
   › A PEEP of up to 5 cmH$_2$O is a reasonable starting point in most patients, although very large patients or those with high oxygen requirements may require higher levels of PEEP.
   › It is worth having a look at the pressure-volume curves on the ventilator and adjusting PEEP to optimise position on the curve for maximum compliance.
   › Short procedures will not require PEEP.
7. Review inspiratory: expiratory ratio
   › This is the ratio of the inspiratory time to expiratory time. It is normally 1:2.
   › Although altered inspiratory: expiratory ratios are more a feature of intensive care ventilation, you need to check that a reasonable ratio has been set!
8. Adjust settings according to physiological parameters
   › Each patient is different and the situation is dynamic; therefore, the ventilator settings need to be adjusted based on indicators of the patient's ventilation (e.g. SpO_2, end-tidal expired CO_2, arterial blood gas analysis, if being measured).

TRANSFER VENTILATORS

When are they used?

Ventilated patients may need to be transferred inside or outside the hospital for a variety of reasons (e.g. to computed tomography scan or to a specialist centre). There are several types of transfer ventilator available and your choice will depend upon:

- what is available
- the condition of the patient (or the level of ventilatory support required)
- the conditions of the transfer (the availability of power supply and oxygen).

What are the main differences?

Ventilators for transfer should be portable and lightweight. They should be relatively easy to operate and may not offer a large variety of different modes. It should be possible to control the tidal volume and pressures delivered to the patient, and to apply PEEP.

During transfer, external power and piped oxygen may not be available, and portable ventilators should therefore offer efficient use of power and oxygen to avoid consumption of supplies.

How is gas supplied?

During a transfer, cylinders usually provide oxygen. It is important to calculate the amount of oxygen that will be required prior to transfer. The control of the oxygen concentration delivered to the patient may be much more limited, and transfer ventilators may only offer settings of '100% oxygen', 'oxygen/air mix', or 'air'. It is not possible to measure the concentration of oxygen being delivered to the patient.

Some ventilators will stop working if the gas supply fails.

How is the power supplied?

Power is usually supplied by a battery, which will have a limited lifespan. The duration of the battery may vary between different ventilators, and also with the ventilator settings. It is important to ensure the battery is fully charged and if possible take a spare battery. You may be able to connect the ventilator to an external power supply once in a transfer vehicle.

What additional safety measures should be undertaken when using transfer ventilators?

It is important to be confident that you are able to operate that specific ventilator. You may not have senior support if you are undertaking the transfer alone. It is useful to have a trial period using the ventilator prior to transfer, to ensure ventilation is adequate for your patient's requirements. Check this with an arterial blood gas analysis.

In case of problems with the ventilator during transfer, an alternative means of ventilating the patient should be available for emergency use. This is normally in the form of a self-inflating bag and an oxygen cylinder.

MINUTE VOLUME DIVIDERS

What is a minute volume divider ventilator?

A minute volume divider ventilator is powered by the gas delivered to it. The total volume of gas delivered to the ventilator each minute will equal the minute volume delivered to the patient. This volume of gas is then divided into preset tidal volumes. The respiratory rate (frequency) will therefore be determined by the selected tidal volume (e.g. for minute volume of 5 L, if tidal volume is set as 500 mL, respiratory rate will be 10).

The minute volume divider functions by two sets of bellows.

Key points

- The reason that you are ventilating the patient will determine the mode of ventilation that you use.
- The adequacy of ventilation is measured by the clearance of CO_2.
- Oxygenation depends upon alveoli being held open. PEEP may improve this.
- Have a systematic approach to setting up a ventilator, ensuring that you set the appropriate alarm limits.
- You must be familiar with the transfer ventilator that your department uses and how to troubleshoot it.

CHAPTER 9

Airway assessment

CHARLOTTE ASH

INTRODUCTION

The difficult airway is defined as 'the clinical situation in which a practitioner experiences difficulty with adequate maintenance and/or protection of the airway'.[1] This can be separated into two categories:

1. difficulty in performing bag-mask ventilation
2. problematic intubation of the trachea.

These are not mutually exclusive and difficulty with ventilation often predicts a challenging intubation. This chapter will provide information on why, when, how and on whom we assess the airway. The majority of the components are easy to cover; how to perform the assessment is more difficult and requires a structured approach.

WHY? THE IMPORTANCE OF ASSESSING THE AIRWAY

It is well known that difficulties in achieving adequate ventilation and failure to secure an airway accounts for significant anaesthetic morbidity and mortality.[2] Historically, up to 28% of deaths in anaesthesia were thought to be caused by failure to intubate or appropriately ventilate the patient.[3]

Correct airway management is the primary role of an anaesthetist. Any simple assessments that can predict challenges in establishing and maintaining an airway prior to intervention can only assist the anaesthetist.

For those patients with an anticipated problematic airway, the 'difficult airway' trolley should be brought to theatre in advance, senior support can be requested, the most appropriate method for securing the airway discussed and a plan made for how to proceed should this initial attempt fail.

WHICH PATIENTS NEED AN AIRWAY ASSESSMENT AND WHEN SHOULD IT BE PERFORMED?

This is simple: all patients coming to theatre for a procedure requiring the involvement of an anaesthetist, regardless of the method of anaesthesia being used, require an airway assessment. For example, a patient listed for a dynamic hip screw fixation under spinal anaesthetic may require an unexpected intubation in the event that spinal anaesthesia is inadequate. All airway assessments should take place during the preoperative assessment.

HISTORY

Prior to clinical examination, a detailed history and thorough review of the patient case notes are vital components in the assessment of any airway. Ask the patient specifically about previous procedures under general anaesthetic including any airway problems experienced. When a patient with a difficult airway is encountered it is valuable to inform the patient of any problems post-operatively. Conversing with a patient also gives an ideal opportunity to assess for hoarseness or stridor. Factors in the history that may be important include:

- Where does the surgeon need to access? This will often influence your choice of endotracheal tube and airway management techniques.
- Does the planned procedure indicate any possible issues regarding calibre of the airway? For example, dental extraction for an abscess may indicate limited mouth opening, or a laser excision of a vocal cord tumour suggests abnormal cords which may make insertion of an endotracheal tube more difficult.

Past medical history

Certain congenital conditions are associated with a difficult airway:

- Down's syndrome
- Pierre Robin's syndrome
- Klippel-Feil's syndrome
- Treacher Collins' syndrome.

Other acquired conditions suggesting possible airway issues include:

- pregnancy
- obesity
- infections (e.g. epiglottitis, croup)
- burns and inhalational injury can result in life-threatening airway oedema
- masses: malignant or benign tumours, cysts, thyroid goitres
- obstructive sleep apnoea
- arthritis of the cervical spine and spondylitis resulting in poor neck mobility
- cervical spine, head or neck trauma
- previous radiotherapy often results in scarring and distorted anatomy
- history of reflux or dyspepsia – this indicates a risk of aspiration of gastric contents and so should be considered in all patients when assessing which airway device is most appropriate.

Past surgical history

- Previous head and neck surgery may indicate swelling, fibrosis and distorted anatomy.
- Previous laryngeal or tracheal procedures may result in tracheal stenosis.

Review of case notes

Anaesthetic charts from previous surgery are invaluable. They should highlight:

- any ventilation or intubation problems encountered

- laryngoscopy grade (discussed later)
- what airway techniques have previously been used and how well these worked.

Your anaesthetic must take into account recent changes in the patient's medical condition. For example, a simple intubation 2 years previously may prove considerably more difficult if the patient has since undergone radiotherapy for a tumour of the larynx.

CLINICAL EXAMINATION

Predicting difficult *ventilation*

Langeron *et al.*[4] in 2000 found a 5% incidence of difficult mask ventilation. Their study also indentified five independent factors for predicting difficult ventilation. The presence of two or more of the following factors indicates a patient is at high risk:

- age >55 years
- history of snoring
- a beard can indicate difficulty achieving a good seal with a face mask
- lack of teeth
- body mass index >26 kg/m².

Other influential factors include:

- restriction of the cervical spine or temporomandibular joint
- facial malformations
- other structural variations including large tongue, large thyroid gland, receding jaw
- concurrent lung disease.

Predicting difficult *intubation*

The incidence of a difficult laryngoscopy or intubation is thought to lie between 1.5% and 13%.[5] Many bedside tests have been introduced to help the anaesthetist identify a possible difficult intubation, yet over half of all cases fail to be anticipated preoperatively.[6] Predicted difficulty with mask ventilation has also been shown to correlate with the occurrence of difficult intubation.[4]

LEMON

Use of the acronym LEMON is helpful when trying to remember important clinical aspects of any airway assessment:

Look at the patient

In particular look for:

- a receding mandible
- prominent, protruding teeth and overbite
- a broad neck
- head and neck masses
- scars, which may indicate previous intervention and any signs of head, neck or chest trauma.

Evaluate the 3-3-2 rule

- Assess the inter-incisor gap by asking the patient to place three fingers vertically between their upper and lower teeth with the mouth maximally open. If this distance is less than 3 cm this implies more difficulty gaining access to the mouth.
- Thyromental distance. This involves assessment of the distance from the thyroid notch to the tip of the jaw or mentum with the mouth closed and the head maximally extended. This represents the position of the larynx from the tongue base. This normally measures >6.5 cm (or more than three finger breadths); a distance of <6 cm indicates a more difficult intubation.[5]

In addition to the 3-3-2 rule, the sternomental distance can also be used. This is measured from the sternum to tip of the mandible with the mouth closed and head extended and predicts a difficult intubation at a distance of 12 cm or less.

Modified Mallampati Classification

This score was first published in 1985[7] and later modified by Samsoon and Young.[8] It involves assigning a score based on the appearance of the oropharynx. The test is performed with the patient sitting with his or her head placed in a neutral position with the mouth fully open and the tongue protruded as far as is possible. The view seen is classified into four categories depending upon which structures are visible:

- Class I: Faucial pillars, soft palate, hard palate and uvula fully visible.
- Class II: All of above, however the tip of uvula is obscured.
- Class III: Soft palate is visible
- Class IV: Soft palate is completely obscured, only hard palate is visible.

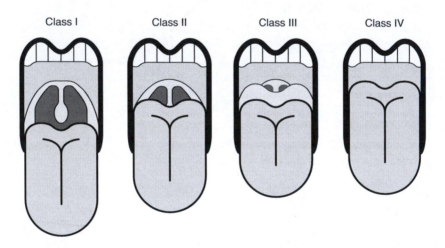

FIGURE 9.1 The Modified Mallampati Classification

In patients with a Mallampati class I appearance, intubation *should* be relatively easy to perform and often correlates to a Grade I view at laryngoscopy (discussed further later). Classes III and IV indicate a difficult intubation. The predicted sensitivity of the Mallampati Test alone lies between 42% and 81% and specificity from 66% to 84%.[5]

Obstruction
- Consider any cause for obstruction – tumour, thyroid goitre, haematoma or foreign body.

Neck mobility
- Flexion of the neck and extension at the atlanto-axial joint is termed the 'sniffing the morning air' position. This is known to provide the best intubating conditions, as it tends to align structures within the neck and provide an optimum view at laryngoscopy. The ability to achieve this position should be tested in all patients (with the exception of those immobilised due to possible or confirmed cervical spine fractures) and is particularly pertinent if there are risk factors for joint or neck immobility. Immobilisation in a hard collar by definition reduces mobility at the neck and is often thought to increase the grade at laryngoscopy.
- Minimum extension should be at least 35 degrees.

ADDITIONAL TESTS
Calder mandibular protrusion test
The patient is asked to protrude the mandible as far forward as possible and a score is assigned.
- Class A: The lower incisors could be protruded anterior to the upper incisors.
- Class B: The lower incisors could be brought into line with the edge of the upper incisors but not anterior.
- Class C: The lower incisors could not be brought in line with the upper incisors.

This test is designed to predict the adequacy of the view at laryngoscopy, class A giving the most favourable conditions.

Wilson's Risk Score
This score assigns a value of 0, 1 or 2 to five defined characteristics (*see* Table 9.1).[9]

TABLE 9.1 Scoring system for Wilson's Risk Score

Characteristic	Score		
	0	1	2
Weight	<90 kg	90–110 kg	>110 kg
Head and neck movement	>90°	~90°	<90°
Jaw movement	IG >5 cm	IG <5 cm	IG <5 cm
	Calder A	Calder B	Calder C
Receding mandible	Normal	Moderate	Severe
Protruding teeth	Normal	Moderate	Severe

IG, incisor gap

A difficult intubation is predicted with a score of 4 or greater.

VIEW AT LARYNGOSCOPY

Although this is not technically a preoperative assessment of the airway, a documented grading of the view at laryngoscopy from previous anaesthetic charts can be extremely useful when forming the anaesthetic plan and deciding when to call for senior support. It is important to remember that a Grade II intubation in experienced hands could prove more difficult for a trainee to achieve.

Cormack and Lehane[10] initially proposed grading of the view at laryngoscopy in 1984. Figure 9.2 shows the structures seen for the four grades. Grades III and IV indicate a difficult intubation.

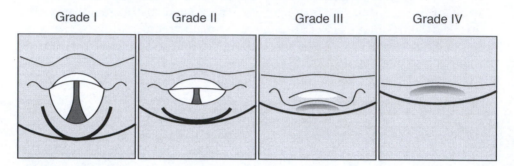

| Grade I | Grade II | Grade III | Grade IV |

FIGURE 9.2 Grading of the view at laryngoscopy

Sensitivity varies greatly between the tests described and is subject to significant user error. They also show a high rate of false-positives – that is, intubations that were predicted to be difficult but were in fact Grade I. The tests mentioned here are most useful in predicting difficult intubations when used in combination; this tends to increase their specificity but decreases sensitivity. Despite your best efforts the unanticipated difficult airway will be encountered, but carefully applying the methods described will reduce this occurrence.

Key points

- A difficult airway describes problems in maintaining an airway, providing ventilation or achieving intubation of the trachea.
- All patients should have an airway assessment, regardless of the type of anaesthesia.
- Perform a detailed history, examination and review of the notes.
- There are various classification systems that aim to predict a difficult airway. They work best when used in combination.
- Grading the laryngoscopy allows others to understand your notes later.

REFERENCES

1. Pearce A. Introduction and definitions. *Curr Anaesth Crit Care.* 2001; **12**(4): 197–200.
2. Caplan RA, Posner KL, Ward RJ, *et al.* Adverse respiratory events in anaesthesia: a closed claims analysis. *Anesthesiology.* 1990; **72**(5): 828–33.

3. Benumof JL. Definition and incidence of difficult airway. In: Benumof JL, editor. *Airway Management: principles and practice*. St Louis: Mosby; 1996. pp. 121–5.
4. Langeron O, Masso E, Huraux C, *et al*. Prediction of difficult mask ventilation. *Anesthesiology*. 2000; **92**(5): 1229–36.
5. Randell T. Prediction of difficult intubation. *Acta Anaesthesiol Scand*. 1996; **40**(8 Pt. 2): 1016–23.
6. Otto CW. Tracheal intubation. In: Nunn JF, Utting JE, Brown BR, editors. *General Anaesthesia*. 5th ed. Boston: Butterworths; 1989. pp. 533–4.
7. Mallampati SR, Gatt SP, Gugino LD, *et al*. A clinical sign to predict difficult tracheal intubation: a prospective study. *Can Anaesth Soc J*. 1985; **32**(4): 429–34.
8. Samsoon GL, Young JR. Difficult tracheal intubation: a retrospective study. *Anaesthesia*. 1987; **42**(5): 487–90.
9. Wilson ME, Spiegelhalter D, Robertson JA, *et al*. Predicting difficult intubation. *Br J Anaesth*. 1988; **61**(2): 211–16.
10. Cormack RS, Lehane J. Difficult tracheal intubation in obstetrics. *Anaesthesia*. 1984; **39**(11): 1105–11.

CHAPTER 10

Airway management

ANDREW DAVIES AND JOHN MOORE

INTRODUCTION

Perhaps the most daunting thing about starting in anaesthesia is that people around you suddenly regard you as 'the airway person'. That's a natural reaction. Until now you may well have managed airways in the injured patient but it's probable that you have never electively removed control of the airway from a fit and well patient.

This chapter cannot possibly explain how to manage the airway of all patients in all situations, but it will describe a logical framework that can be followed for most patients coming to the operating theatre, turning a daunting situation into a very satisfying one.

To get the most out of this chapter, read it in combination with a good equipment book and then the next operating that list you have ask to talk through airway management with the consultant. You will be able to use this chapter to generate a discussion about airway management in different situations (undoubtedly they will not agree with everything here!) and will be able to handle the equipment described.

AIRWAY AXIOMS

Here are a few things that must always be in mind before you take control of someone's airway.

- Always assess the airway before you interfere with it (*see* Chapter 9).
- Hand ventilation by face mask is the most important skill to acquire. Inability to intubate the trachea is not a problem if you can do this.
- Failure to oxygenate kills patients, not failure to intubate.
- Failure to plan for failure is a common source of problems: always have fallback airway management plans.
- Never be afraid to wake the patient up.

AIRWAY CONTROL TECHNIQUES

There are a variety of tools and techniques employed by anaesthetists to hold open the airway. This text can't serve as a full guide to all the equipment available: for that it is strongly recommended that you read a good equipment book in combination with hands-on experience of the devices.

How to choose which of these techniques is appropriate for your patient followed by descriptions of these techniques are described next.

CHOOSING AN AIRWAY

This is the system we use to decide which of the airway control techniques to employ. It is based on three questions:

1. What did the airway assessment show?
    > Is it a proven difficult airway (i.e. there has been a difficult intubation in the past) or a likely difficult airway? This will mean a requirement for special equipment if intubation is required and maybe an awake fibreoptic intubation if there is a full stomach.
    > A normal/easy airway? This means that any airway device can be used depending on the answers to the following two questions.
2. Does the patient have a full stomach or its equivalent?
    > If yes, then the airway needs to be secured with an endotracheal tube (ETT) to prevent pulmonary aspiration of gastric contents. This will generally mandate rapid sequence induction (RSI) or, if in combination with a difficult airway, awake fibreoptic intubation.
3. What is the planned operation?
    > The duration and nature of the operation will have a bearing on airway choice as will the required position of the patient to allow surgical access (*see* Table 10.1)

Here are worked examples covering the majority of common situations.

Normal airway, empty stomach/no reflux

- The majority of elective patients will be in this category: a normal airway that doesn't preclude face mask or laryngeal mask airway (LMA) so the airway management decision rests on the type and duration of operation being planned (*see* Table 10.1).

Normal airway but full stomach / risk of reflux

- A standard scenario for emergency surgical patients (e.g. those presenting with appendicitis).
- Here RSI is the technique of choice.

Difficult airway, no risk of reflux

- Once again the airway depends to some extent on the planned operation. If this allows for LMA or face mask anaesthetic, be prepared for difficulty and failure / conversion to intubation.
- If the operation requires the patient to be intubated then there are a variety of techniques one could employ:
    > intravenous induction, intubation using difficult airway adjuncts (e.g. flexible fibreoptic laryngoscope, rigid videolaryngoscope, intubating LMA)
    > gas induction and then direct or fibreoptic laryngoscopy and intubation.

Difficult airway, high risk of reflux

- Awake fibreoptic intubation is the safest technique, although this should be carried out under the supervision of a senior anaesthetist, especially if required for emergency surgery.

FACE MASK ANAESTHETIC

Mastering face mask technique should be the primary goal of every novice to anaesthesia. Sadly, you probably won't get to conduct many operations just on a face mask as the LMA has become its almost ubiquitous replacement for even the quickest procedures. This is a shame as one of the benefits of face mask anaesthesia is that it keeps you connected to the patient at all time and allows you to function as a very sensitive monitor: you will be able to feel if the airway starts to obstruct or if the patient develops a degree of laryngospasm.

TABLE 10.1 Operative factors determining airway selection

Operative factors	Airway
'Body cavity surgery' Abdominal surgery, neurosurgery, thoracic surgery	ETT
Shared airway Oral and dental surgery, some ENT procedures	ETT Some situations may require a nasal ETT to allow the surgeon adequate access
'Distant airway' (i.e. when the patient's airway becomes inaccessible because of draping or positioning, e.g. prone or shoulder surgery)	ETT
Surgical duration >1 hour	ETT, LMA (not recommended, but possible)
Non–body cavity, duration <1 hour	Face mask or LMA

ENT, ear, nose and throat; ETT, endotracheal tube; LMA, laryngeal mask airway

To this end we would advise that you actively ask the consultant with whom you're working if you can conduct any quick cases on the list using a face mask. This will make you stand out immediately as someone who has already grasped the fundamental lesson of airway control and is as keen as mustard.

FACE MASK TECHNIQUE

- Face mask technique is best learned from an expert.
- With your little finger under the angle of the jaw place your ring and middle fingers onto the bone of the mandible and bring your thumb and forefinger over the top of the face mask to make a 'c' shape. This will enable you to perform a jaw thrust, chin lift and apply gentle downward pressure on the mask creating a gas-tight seal.
- You may need an oropharyngeal airway.
- With your other hand you can write the chart and make any adjustments to the anaesthetic machine that are necessary.

- Practise holding the face mask with each hand independently – the anaesthetic machine may not always be on the same side!
- A two-handed technique is sometimes required.

SUPRAGLOTTIC AIRWAY DEVICES

There is an ever-expanding multitude of devices designed to sit in the pharynx immediately above the glottis through which a patient may breathe under anaesthesia. The original was the LMA.

The main use of these devices should be in spontaneously breathing patients for procedures lasting less than an hour. You will see them used in a variety of other situations including with patients paralysed and ventilated but you can't go wrong if you stick to the mantra of spontaneously breathing for less than 60 minutes.

Laryngeal mask airway technique

- Induction of anaesthesia either intravenously or via the inhalational route. Propofol is an excellent induction agent for insertion of the LMA.
- Place the patient's head into the 'sniffing the morning air' position and get your assistant to perform a jaw thrust.
- Insert the LMA gently into the mouth following the curvature of the hard palate; you will feel it 'drop' into the correct position.
- Inflate the cuff and then check airway patency – if spontaneously breathing you should see smooth chest and bag movement and appropriate capnography. If the patient is not spontaneously breathing then gently squeeze the bag on the breathing circuit: the chest should rise smoothly with minimal resistance and there should be a normal capnograph trace.

ENDOTRACHEAL INTUBATION

This section will deal with oral endotracheal intubation. There are some general principles:

- always check all equipment before starting, ensuring that you have the correct range and sizes of face masks, LMAs, laryngoscopes, tubes, and powerful suction
- check the anaesthetic machine
- ensure the patient has full monitoring attached
- ensure you have discussed the plan you intend to follow with your anaesthetic assistant and your plans in case of failure.

TRACHEAL INTUBATION IN PATIENTS WITHOUT RISK OF ASPIRATION

- Induce anaesthesia: gas or intravenous induction. There exists controversy over the practice of so-called 'check' ventilation (i.e. checking that one can ventilate the patient using the face mask prior to administration of muscle relaxant). The theory of this technique is that if you feel unable to ventilate the patient one would not paralyse the patient and then run the risk of a 'can't intubate, can't ventilate' scenario. Suffice to say that some people use this technique and others don't. Thankfully, a 'can't intubate, can't ventilate' scenario is incredibly rare.
- Depending on the choice of muscle relaxant it may be up to 3 minutes before adequate intubating conditions are gained. During this time one maintains

anaesthesia using volatile agents or 'total intravenous anaesthesia' and one maintains ventilation of the lungs via a face mask.

- Head positioning is absolutely critical to success and a pillow is a crucial tool. Position so that the head is in the 'sniffing the morning air' position. Sometimes two pillows are required to achieve this.
- Select laryngoscope blade: a size 3.0 Macintosh blade is sufficient for most adults. Some males will require a size 4.0 blade.
- Select ETT size – a size 7.0–8.0 for most women and 8.0–9.0 for most men.
- Holding the laryngoscope in your left hand, carefully insert the blade into the mouth. Aim for the right tonsil and then sweep into the midline, pushing the tongue over to the left. Once you can see the epiglottis continue advancing the blade into the vallecula. Lift the laryngoscope in the direction of the long axis of the handle as you do so the epiglottis will be levered upward and the glottis will fall beautifully into view. *Do not lever* the laryngoscope against the teeth: this will lead to dental damage.
- If you don't get a good view try pressure on the neck with your right hand: if this pushes the larynx into view get your assistant to continue the pressure there.
- Take hold of the ETT at the proximal tip. Hold it lightly; it should have a natural curve that will follow the hard palate with ease. If you hold it in the middle the tube will bend, pushing the tip downward and making placement through the rima glottidis more difficult.
- Pass the tube through the glottis being observant of the tube markings: the aim is to be mid-tracheal, which in an adult is at around 18–24 cm from the teeth.
- Your assistant will inflate the ETT cuff while you gently ventilate – ensure there is the minimum amount of air in the cuff needed to create a seal.
- Check there is a good capnograph trace with an adequate plateau phase to confirm that you are not in the oesophagus, then auscultate both sides of the chest in the axillae, listening for equal bilateral air entry, to ensure the tube has not been placed into the right (or, unusually, left) main bronchus.
- Secure the tube to the patient using ties or tape; keep a close eye at this time that the tube doesn't get pushed in further: if in doubt reassess by auscultation.
- If laryngoscopy is good but placement is difficult a gum-elastic bougie may be useful: this can be placed through the glottis and then an ETT railroaded over the top.
- Throughout this whole process be mindful that you aren't ventilating the patient and that the patient will start to desaturate if you take a long time to intubate: there should never be a rush to intubate in this group of patients. If you are unable to pass the tube, reventilate the patient for a minute or two while moving to the next stage of your airway plan. Ensure optimal positioning and then decide what you need for success at the next attempt. If you are having difficulty, always remember: call for help early if you are on your own and you can always wake the patient up (depending on time since muscle relaxant administered and type of relaxant).

Rapid sequence induction
- The purpose of RSI is to induce anaesthesia and then secure the airway in as

short a time as is safe, thus limiting the time when aspiration of gastric contents could occur.

- You must explain to the patient what will happen: that they will be pre-oxygenated with a face mask and then cricoid pressure will be applied as they go to sleep.
- Cricoid pressure is pressure of 30 N applied to the cricoid ring. This should be sufficient to press the oesophagus closed against the spine. This theoretically creates a mechanical barrier to reflux of gastric contents into the oropharynx. Also called Sellick's manoeuvre after the British anaesthetist who pioneered its use.
- Start by preparing your drugs. For RSI the classical combination would be induction with thiopentone and relaxation with suxamethonium, calculate the amount you are going to give in advance. The logic of this choice is that they are both short-acting so in the event of failure to intubate, the patient will awaken quickly, regaining control of his or her own airway and removing the risk of aspiration.
- Pre-oxygenate: the purpose of this manoeuvre is to remove all the air from the lungs, or, more specifically, to denitrogenate the lungs. The entire functional residual capacity is now filled with oxygen, thus allowing up to 8 minutes' apnoea before desaturation occurs. Apply a well-fitting face mask gently to the patient's face; a gas-tight seal is essential. Allow the patient to breathe 100% oxygen for 3 minutes. Monitor the end-tidal oxygen concentration during this time – the goal is >85%.
- An alternative method is to get the patient to take three to five vital capacity breaths.
- Have a powerful sucker to hand (i.e. under the pillow and turned on) in case of aspiration.
- Begin induction, instruct assistant to begin cricoid pressure once you have decided the patient is anaesthetised. Administer suxamethonium.
- Wait for 1 minute, or for the termination of fasciculation, and then attempt laryngoscopy.
- Some authors advocate gentle ventilation with 100% oxygen while waiting for the suxamethonium to work. The risk is that you could inflate the stomach, making regurgitation even more likely.
- Laryngoscopy and intubation should then take place as described earlier. It is worth noting that cricoid pressure can distort laryngeal anatomy if inexpertly applied. In addition, the assistant's hand applying cricoid pressure can obstruct placement of the laryngoscope into the mouth: especially so in obstetric patients who have enlarged breasts.
- It is important to remember that the key to RSI is prevention of aspiration, thus if you have unanticipated difficulty in intubation early abandonment and waking the patient must be at the forefront of your mind.
- Once intubated, inflate the tube cuff and confirm tube position with capnography. If the tube is endotracheal instruct the assistant to release cricoid pressure. Check and tie the tube as described earlier.
- Maintain anaesthesia by whatever method you have planned.

Awake fibreoptic intubation

- Awake fibreoptic intubation is an advanced technique that is beyond the scope of this book; however, it is useful to understand it as a concept.
- For patients who are known, or strongly suspected, to be a difficult intubation and who may also have risk factors for gastric aspiration or other factors precluding asleep attempts at intubation.
- The patient is awake and the airway is anaesthetised topically with local anaesthetic by a variety of methods or by nerve blocks.
- The patient is intubated using a fibreoptic scope with a pre-loaded ETT on the scope.
- Once intubation is confirmed, general anaesthesia is commenced and then the cuff of the ETT is inflated.

EXTUBATION

Extubation is often forgotten but it is just as important as intubation. A large proportion of airway disasters occur at extubation when your guard is down. Some institutions allow trained recovery nurses to extubate patients in recovery without direct supervision by an anaesthetist. As a novice to anaesthesia it is important that every patient that you intubate you also extubate, so that you become proficient in this skill.

EXTUBATION FOLLOWING AN EASY AIRWAY WITH NO ASPIRATION RISK

- Here extubation should be as calm and as straightforward as intubation was.
- The options are to extubate awake or deep.
- Deep extubation involves allowing the patient to start breathing spontaneously while still deeply anaesthetised and then suctioning out any secretions in the mouth, smoothly extubating the patient and then holding the airway open using a face mask and switching off the anaesthetic, allowing the patient to wake.
- The advantage is that the patient's airway reflexes are still dulled so the tube can be removed without causing coughing; this is beneficial in neurosurgery and ophthalmic surgery where raises in intracranial and intraocular pressure are to be avoided.
- Doing this with the patient in too light a plane of anaesthesia will result in laryngospasm and coughing and may necessitate emergency re-intubation.
- The more common method is to extubate patients awake. Here the anaesthetic is stopped and the patient is ventilated until he or she starts breathing.
- Before the patient becomes too light suction out all secretions from the mouth and oropharynx that might otherwise irritate the larynx.
- If a muscle relaxant has been utilised it must be adequately reversed and the patient extubated only when the patient can stick out his or her tongue (indicating airway control) or lift his or her head off the pillow for 5 seconds (indicating muscle power has returned).
- Once you have decided that the patient is ready to be extubated get the patient to open his or her mouth widely and smoothly pull out the tube while applying positive pressure to the bag (to blow any secretions off the vocal cords).
- Post-extubation transfer to recovery and monitor closely.

EXTUBATION AFTER A RAPID SEQUENCE INDUCTION OR A DIFFICULT INTUBATION

- Here deep extubation is *not* an option, as the patient will be at risk of aspiration or loss of airway.
- Patients are extubated according to the awake system outlined earlier but also placed left-lateral and slightly head-down to prevent aspiration of vomitus.

At the time of writing, the Difficult Airway Society is drawing up guidelines for extubation: it is well worth checking the society's website to see the latest guidance (www. das.uk.com).

THE UNANTICIPATED DIFFICULT AIRWAY

There is, alas, no perfect system to predict difficult laryngoscopy or difficult intubation. For this reason it behoves all anaesthetists to stay vigilant and to have plans for failure ready in mind. Difficulty can occur in several scenarios and you should review the Difficult Airway Society Guidelines for management of difficulty in routine intubation, RSI and 'can't intubate, can't ventilate' scenarios. It is well worth memorising these.

These guidelines can be found online (www.das.uk.com/guidelines/downloads. html) and in Appendices 5 and 6.

Key points

- Airway management can be the most rewarding, the most technically challenging and the most frightening part of anaesthesia.
- The ability to hold an airway open with a face mask is paramount.
- Careful assessment of the patient will mean that there are very few incidences of unanticipated difficulty.

FURTHER READING

- Davey AJ, Diba A. *Ward's Anaesthetic Equipment*. 6th ed. London: Elsevier Health Sciences; 2012.
- Fourth National Audit Project of the Royal College of Anaesthetists and the Difficult Airway Society. *Major complications of Airway Management in the UK*. London: The Royal College of Anaesthetists; 2011.
- www.das.uk.com/guidelines/downloads.html

CHAPTER 11

Basic patient positioning

DANIEL COTTLE, RUTH NICHOLSON, KATIE CARDEN AND DANIEL FLAHERTY

Once you have rendered a patient unconscious, you are responsible for that patient's safety during his or her most vulnerable time. It is your job to protect the patient and you should lead all patient positioning.

Your most important considerations are:

- protecting the eyes
- ensuring that the endotracheal tube and intravenous lines stay in place
- preventing diathermy burns
- preventing soft tissue damage
- preventing stretch or compression injury of nerves.

GENERAL POINTS

The eyes must be closed and covered during anaesthesia. If left uncovered they can dry out and corneal abrasions form. Abrasions are also caused by direct contact. Eye ointment may also be used in high-risk cases. Ensure that you use low-adhesive tape and remove it carefully at the end of the case. The eyes are also at risk of direct damage

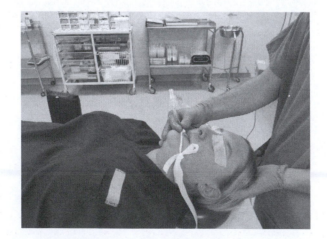

FIGURE 11.1 Holding the head and the tracheal tube in place

during the surgery and you should ensure that there is no equipment (including ventilator tubing) that may cause compression. This can (rarely) lead to ocular venous thrombosis and blindness.

You should hold the endotracheal tube every time the patient is moved and all movements should be authorised by you. Hold it with your hand resting on the patient's cheek to ensure control of the head and the tube.

If the surgeon is using monopolar diathermy, the electrical energy is dissipated through a rectangular metal pad, usually on the leg. If any other part of the patient comes in contact with earthed-metal then this will form the exit point and burning can occur. Ensure that no part of the patient (particularly a limb) is in contact with metal that could form an exit site. You should also ensure that the diathermy pad is positioned away from any internal metal work.

THE SUPINE POSITION

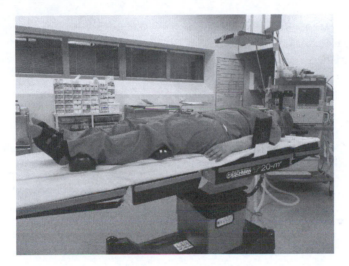

FIGURE 11.2 The supine position

The supine position is by for the most common position that you will use. The biggest risks are to the eyes, compression damage to soft tissues and nerve injury. Be particularly vigilant for the brachial plexus and the ulnar nerve.

Ensure that the head is in a neutral position in order to prevent stretching the brachial plexus (*see* Figure 11.3). Even gentle pressure sustained over a long time can injure an anaesthetised patient. Prevent ventilator tubing resting on patients, especially when the head is covered by drapes. If the head is covered it should be checked regularly.

The arms must be supported at the side of the operating table, especially those of large patients. The ulnar nerve is at risk of compression injury. Padding should be used and the support should be placed across the elbow (*see* Figure 11.4).

During long cases you may need to flex the patient's knees slightly. This prevents stretching of the femoral and popliteal nerves. The knees should also be supported if they have a fixed-flexion deformity to prevent pressure sores on the ankles (*see* Figure 11.5).

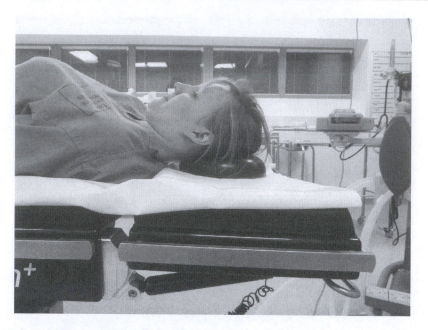

FIGURE 11.3 Maintain the head in a neutral position

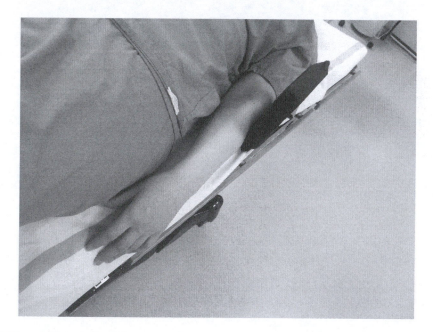

FIGURE 11.4 The arm board

The ankles can also be supported during long cases. If ankle supports are used then the knees must also be supported in flexion to prevent stretching the popliteal nerve.

It maybe useful to have an arm out to the side of the operating table during a case in order to allow you access to your lines. In this position the brachial plexus is at risk

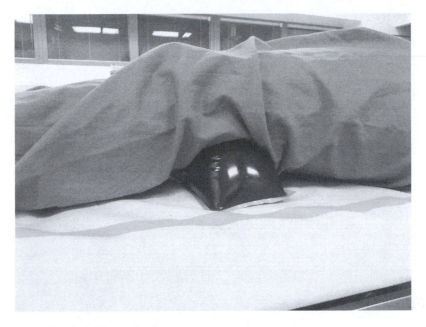

FIGURE 11.5 A gel pad flexes the knees

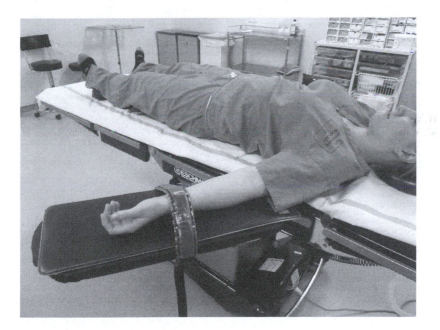

FIGURE 11.6 The arm out at the side

of damage through being stretched. The arm shouldn't be abducted by greater than 90 degrees. You should feel under the arm and over the clavicle for tension in the tissues overlying the plexus. A gel pad provides greater cushioning for the ulnar nerve and the arm should be secured to prevent it falling (*see* Figure 11.6).

THE LITHOTOMY POSITION

The upper body positioning is the same as the supine position. The legs are placed in gutters and raised with the hips and knees flexed. The bottom end of the table is then removed to allow the surgeon access to the pelvis. Damage can occur to the joints, with compression of the femoral and peroneal nerves and stretching of the sciatic.

The legs should be lifted and raised simultaneously. Over-flexion should be avoided and the calf should be felt for compression. There is a risk of compartment syndrome during very long cases.

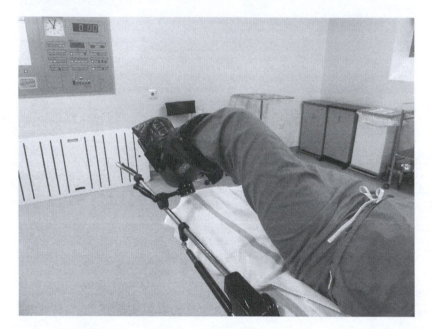

FIGURE 11.7 A single leg placed into the lithotomy position – there must be no compression of the nerves in the calf

THE LATERAL POSITION

The lateral position is used mainly for orthopaedic surgery. The brachial plexus and ulnar nerve are at risk (*see* Figure 11.8). There is compression of the lower arm and you must ensure that the lower shoulder is pulled through. You should place intravenous access in the upper arm as venous hypertension in the lower arm may prevent the drip running and risks extravasation.

The lower arm should have the shoulder pulled through and the elbow flexed. This should be supported with an arm board, being careful not to compress the ulnar nerve.

The upper arm is placed in a gutter. Check the axillary and the supraclavicular tissues for stretching of the brachial plexus and prevent compression of the median nerve as the arm enters the gutter (*see* Figure 11.9).

Supports are placed on the anterior superior iliac spine and the lumbar lordosis. Ensure that the former are over the bone crest and not compressing the femoral nerve or vessels. A pillow between the legs prevents adduction of the thigh and compression damage at the ankles.

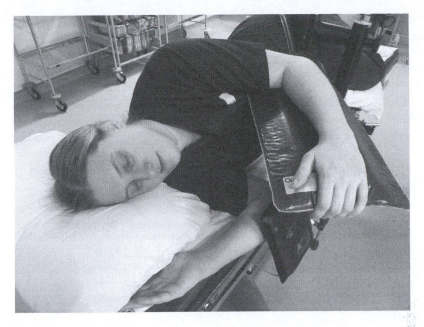

FIGURE 11.8 The lateral position

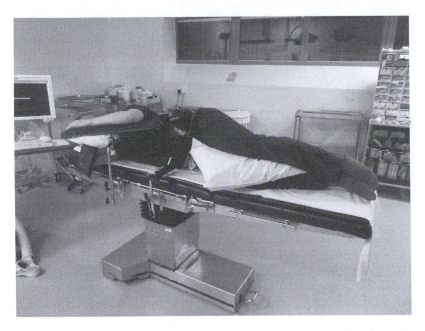

FIGURE 11.9 The superior arm is in the gutter while the inferior arm is flexed and free of the body

THE PRONE POSITION

The prone position is a complicated position that carries a high risk of ocular, nerve and soft tissue damage if it is not performed correctly. It is beyond the scope of this book and you should not perform it unless you have been trained to do so.

> **Key points**
> - Patient positioning increases in complexity and you will need to have face-to-face training.
> - You must ensure that the tracheal tube, intravenous lines and monitoring devices remain in position when you transfer a patient.
> - Carefully protect the eyes and all peripheral nerve pressure points.

CHAPTER 12

Recovery, handover and protocols

JASBIR CHHABRA

THE OBJECTIVES OF A RECOVERY ROOM

Recovery rooms began less than 50 years ago when it was realised that early post-operative morbidity and mortality were preventable if specialised nursing care was available in the immediate post-operative period. With an increase in complex surgical procedures in an increasingly ageing population with multiple co-morbidities, recovery room care was extended beyond the first few hours after surgery to overnight recovery rooms. This eventually led to the development of level II care facilities for post-operative patients.

The main objective of post-anaesthetic care is to have an awake, cooperative and comfortable patient who is maintaining his or her airway, is well oxygenated and is cardiovascularly stable.

HANDOVER

The anaesthetist should transfer the patient from the theatre to the recovery room ensuring adequate monitoring and support.

Following the transfer of the patient to the recovery room, good handover and clear instructions to the recovery staff responsible for the patient helps predict and avoid common problems encountered in the recovery room.

A good handover provides clear documentation and verbal communication of the:

- patient's details including co-morbid conditions
- operative procedure performed
- the site of surgery
- the anaesthetic technique including the use of regional anaesthesia
- any problems in the intra-operative period including blood loss
- anticipated post-operative problems
- clear post-operative instructions for recovery as well as for post-operative care on the ward.

While communicating the anaesthetic technique one should explain the type of anaesthesia, the analgesic agents used and prophylaxis of post-operative nausea and vomiting. For major procedures it is good practice to hand over the input output balance in terms of the amount of fluids and blood products used and the total urine output during surgery.

It is mandatory for the anaesthetist to be available while the patient is still in recovery.

ROUTINE CARE IN THE RECOVERY AREA

- On arrival of the patient in the recovery area, an assessment is made of the patient's:
  > consciousness level
  > airway
  > breathing (respiratory rate and pulse oximetry)
  > circulation (pulse rate, blood pressure and electrocardiograph monitoring)
  > temperature.
- After receiving a handover the recovery nurse then examines the wound site and drains for any excessive bleeding.
- All patients after general anaesthesia receive 30%–40% oxygen during emergence.
- Vital signs are monitored based on protocol but usually every 5 minutes for 15 minutes or until stable and then every 15 minutes thereafter.
- Once the patient is fully conscious, assessment of patient comfort and post-operative pain control is established.
- When prescribed, recovery nurses administer boluses of intravenous opioids or patient controlled analgesia.
- Those at risk of hypoxia, including those on opioids, should be prescribed oxygen according to local protocols for the recovery period and the ward.
- The patient should be nursed in the head-up position (when possible) to optimise oxygenation.
- Following regional anaesthesia, sensory and motor levels should be measured and recorded. The presence of motor block should be recorded.

COMMON PROBLEMS IN THE RECOVERY AREA

Many problems that arise in the recovery room can be anticipated based on the patient's co-morbidities, the surgical procedure and the intra-operative course. For example, a morbidly obese patient with sleep apnoea and coexisting hypertension who has had an ear, nose and throat procedure, is at risk of post-operative airway obstruction and type II respiratory failure.

The main problems can be classified into the following categories.

Airway

- The patient may be at risk of compromising or obstructing his airway in the recovery room due to the residual effect of the anaesthetic agents (relaxed soft tissues of the pharynx), sedatives and opioids.
- Obstruction may also be due to:
  > blood or secretions
  > dentures
  > vomit
  > a foreign body.

- Pre-existing airway problems as well as upper airway surgery can increase the risk further.

Good assessment of the airway maintenance and patency is very important in the post-operative period. Both you and the recovery nurse ought to be well versed with simple airway manoeuvres like a head tilt chin lift and jaw thrust, and in the use of airway adjuncts like oropharyngeal and nasopharyngeal airway to maintain a patent airway.

Breathing
- Breathing may be affected by:
  - › a compromised airway
  - › the residual effects of anaesthetic agents, opioids and muscle relaxants
  - › co-morbidities like chronic obstructive pulmonary disease and asthma
  - › a distended abdomen
  - › post-operative pain reducing respiratory and cough effort.

'Look, listen and feel' is a very good way to assess a patient's breathing. Use of pulse oximetry and arterial blood gases also help in the assessment of oxygenation and adequacy of breathing. Early recognition of compromised breathing and treatment of its causes can help prevent catastrophic consequences.

Circulation
- Common circulatory problems in the recovery room are hypotension, hypertension and arrhythmias.
- The patient's co-morbid conditions, the surgical procedure and the intra-operative course can help you anticipate and prevent problems.
- The most important cause of hypovolaemia (and so hypotension) is bleeding and this should be excluded first. Also consider fluid and electrolyte losses.
- Neuro-axial blockade and vasodilating drugs also cause hypotension.
- Post-operative monitoring of colour, heart rate, blood pressure, capillary refill time, electrocardiograph, mental status and urine output help diagnose post-operative circulatory failure.

Conscious level
- The return of consciousness following general anaesthesia can take some time and can be variable and relapsing.
- A delayed return of consciousness should prompt you to look for the underlying cause. Consider:
  - › the residual effect of anaesthetic agents
  - › hypothermia
  - › hypoglycaemia
  - › hypothyroidism
  - › perioperative stroke
  - › increasing age
  - › obesity.
- Assessment of the conscious level should be based on the AVPU scale

(alert, responsive to a verbal stimulus, responsive to a painful stimulus and unresponsive) or the Glasgow Coma Scale. Also measure pupillary size and responsiveness.

POST-OPERATIVE PAIN

Pain can be self-reported or it can manifest as tachycardia, hypertension and agitation. Knowledge and experience of the degree of pain relief required for a given surgical procedure can help prevent inadequate analgesia. It is important to realise that each patient has a different pain threshold and tolerance and that there is a wide variation in the analgesic requirement of individuals for the same operative procedure (*see* Chapter 13 for treatment strategies).

POST-OPERATIVE NAUSEA AND VOMITING

Post-operative nausea and vomiting is a common problem following general anaesthesia, and it may also result from hypotension following spinal and epidural anaesthesia.
- Risk factors are previous post-operative nausea and vomiting, motion sickness, female sex and non-smokers.
- Opioids, volatile anaesthetic gases and nitrous oxide also cause it.
- Surgical factors include intraperitoneal, squint, gynaecological and middle ear surgery.
- Commonly used antiemetics include ondansetron, dexamethasone, cylizine and propofol infusion.
- *See* Chapter 17.

POST-OPERATIVE SHIVERING AND HYPOTHERMIA

Post-operative shivering is commonly observed as a result of hypothermia following heat loss during anaesthesia. It can also be caused by general and neuro-axial anaesthesia directly.
- A cold ambient temperature in the theatre, the prolonged exposure of large internal body surface areas and un-warmed intravenous fluids can all lead to hypothermia and post-operative shivering.
- Shivering represents the body's effort to increase heat production and raised body temperature. The patient may shiver before the core body temperature has dropped.
- The routine monitoring of core body temperature in the recovery room enables quick diagnosis and warrants the use of warming devices to raise the body temperature to normal. The most common are intravenous fluid warmers and warm air blankets.
- Small intravenous doses of pethidine 10–50 mg can dramatically reduce or even stop shivering but should not be used if the patient is hypothermic.

DISCHARGE CRITERIA

It is important to realise that the criteria for discharging patients from the recovery area can vary according to whether the patient is going to be discharged to an intensive care unit, a regular ward or day case surgery. Use of a discharge protocol ensures uniformity of training, assessment and safe discharge of patients. The discharge of the patient from the recovery unit is the prime responsibility of the anaesthetist, but surgical considerations might mean that the responsibility is shared with the surgeon.

All theatre units should have clear criteria for discharge based on the AAGBI guidelines. These will include:

- an awake and responsive patient who is maintaining his or her own airway
- adequate analgesia
- a stable cardiovascular system
- normal respiration and adequate oxygenation
- normothermia
- no continuing surgical problems (bleeding or drain loss)
- instructions for the ward staff and safe prescriptions for oxygen, drugs and fluid.

Key points

- Recovery rooms play an important role in minimising the morbidity and mortality of patients in the immediate post-operative period.
- Good preoperative assessment, anaesthetic management and surgery prevent problems. You should anticipate problems, which may arise in the immediate post-operative period, and ensure good post-operative instructions for the recovery nurse and the ward staff.
- Good handover and good communication between the recovery nurse and the anaesthetists and surgeons can help minimise many problems in the recovery room.

FURTHER READING

- Association of Anaesthetists of Great Britain and Ireland. Immediate post-anaesthesia recovery 2013. *Anaesthesia*. 2013; **66**(3): 288–97.
- Foster P. Basic anaesthetic training manual, Chapter 10: Postoperative care of the patient. In: *Health and Development Issue 8* (CD-ROM). St Albans, Herts: TALC, 2006. Available at: www.talcuk.org/cd-roms/e-talc-health-and-development-issue-8.htm (accessed 1 June 2013).
- Allman K. Monitoring in the recovery room. *Update in Anaesthesia*.2000; **11**(9). Available at: http://update.anaesthesiologists.org/2000/06/01/monitoring-in-the-recovery-room/ (accessed 1 June 2013).
- King M. Safe recovery from anaesthesia: care before, during and after the operation. In: Ayim E, *et al. Primary Anaesthesia*. New York: Oxford University Press; 1986. pp. 15–22.

CHAPTER 13

Post-operative analgesia

CRISTIAN SALBATICU AND AMANDA SHAW

GENERAL CONSIDERATIONS[1,2,3]

It is the duty of the anaesthetist to provide and prescribe analgesia, especially for the immediate post-operative period. There should also be an anticipation of the required pain relief for the intermediate and long-term period. The surgical team will review the pain requirements on a daily basis, but it will take up to 24 hours until that review takes place. In day case surgery you might have to prescribe the take-home medication.

Post-operative pain relief should be planned before surgery starts and should be discussed and agreed with the patient. The patient is usually anxious not only about the operation ahead but also about the recovery period. Providing a plan for post-operative analgesia might help relieve some of that anxiety.

There is evidence that adequate analgesia results in a quicker recovery, a shorter hospital stay and a reduced incidence of chronic pain. Pain causes an increased sympathetic response, with subsequent tachycardia and increased myocardial oxygen consumption. It also contributes to a reduced mobility, thus increasing the incidence of pneumonia and of thromboembolic events.

There are various ways of providing adequate levels of analgesia, all having advantages and disadvantages.[4] Some may prefer giving a larger dose of analgesic just before the end of the operation; others might wait until the patient is able to communicate and give a dose should there be any pain.

- In the first scenario post-operative pain might be less but at the expense of possible side effects and treating some patients who would otherwise be pain-free.
- In the latter there is the advantage of targeting only those patients in pain and minimising side effects, but at the expense of having some of the patients in pain.

When indicated, some might perform peripheral nerve blockade or ask the surgeons to inject local anaesthetic in the wound (either at the beginning or at the end of the operation). All these interventions usually provide good levels of post-operative analgesia but are associated with their own risks.

Irrespective of the approach used, the most important thing is to have a plan and to be flexible enough to alter it should it fail.

HOW IS PAIN ASSESSED?

Pain is a very personal experience and its interpretation can be subjective. Different pain assessment scales are used to quantify it and their use ensures that everyone looking after the patient 'speaks the same language'.[2]

Facial expressions
- A series of pictograms with different expressions, ranging from happy to tearful.
- These are very useful in patients who cannot communicate (children, elderly, those who do not speak the language).

Verbal scale
- The pain may be rated as none, mild, moderate, severe or very severe.

Numerical scale
- The pain is rated on a scale ranging from 0 to 10, where 0 means no pain and 10 is the worst pain ever.

SIMPLE ANALGESIA[1,2,3,4,5]

Paracetamol[6]
- Has analgesic, antipyretic and weak anti-inflammatory effects
- Used to treat mild to moderate pain
- Can be administered orally (90% bioavailability), rectally (50%–70% bioavailability) or intravenously (100% bioavailability)
- Is more effective when taken on a regular rather than on an 'as required' basis
- Usual dose 1 g 4 to 6 hourly, up to 4 g per 24 hours
- Intravenous preparation can be as efficacious as 10 mg of intramuscular morphine
- Peak effect in 60 minutes (orally); with the intravenous preparation, this occurs at the end of the 15 minute infusion; the rectal route does not achieve peak effect until 2–3 hours following administration
- Overdose can result in hepatic toxicity
- When given together with a weak opioid it provides good analgesia
- Can reduce opioid requirements if given as part of a multimodal analgesia regimen following some types of surgery

NON-STEROIDAL ANTI-INFLAMMATORY DRUGS
- Have anti-inflammatory, antipyretic and weak central analgesic effects
- Often used for their opioid sparing effects
- More potent for bone and muscle pain
- Contraindicated in:
  - history of peptic ulcer or gastrointestinal bleeding
  - cardiac failure (severe)
  - dehydration, hypovolaemia, hypotension
  - surgery with high risk of bleeding (advisable to check with surgeon)
  - pregnancy – the last trimester.

- Caution in:
  - › renal impairment
  - › hepatic impairment
  - › cardiac failure (impaired cardiac function)
  - › asthma (usually not more than 10% of asthmatics are affected)
  - › breastfeeding
  - › pregnancy
  - › interactions with other medications – for example, anticoagulants, selective serotonin reuptake inhibitors and venlafaxine (increased risk of bleeding).

Ibuprofen

- The most commonly used non-steroidal anti-inflammatory drug, ibuprofen has the lowest reported incidence of side effects
- Usual dose is 400 mg 8 hourly (dose can be increased to 2.4 g per 24 hours, seek senior advice)

Diclofenac

- Usual oral dose is 50 mg 8 hourly
- Can be given rectally (50–100 mg suppository)
- An intravenous preparation is available, but it's highly irritant and needs to be diluted and given slowly

Ketorolac

- Potent analgesic with weak anti-inflammatory effect
- Usual dose is 10–30 mg (30 mg has similar potency to 10 mg morphine)
- Reduce the dose in elderly or frail patients

OPIOID ANALGESICS[1,2,3,4,5,7]

- Useful for visceral pain
- Side effects of opioids include:
  - › sedation
  - › nausea and vomiting
  - › vasodilatation and myocardial depression
  - › pruritus
  - › delayed gastric emptying
  - › constipation
  - › urinary retention.
- Routes of opioid administration:
  - › oral – absorption can be reduced by delayed gastric emptying
  - › intranasal – can be useful for children
  - › subcutaneous and transdermal – useful for chronic pain relief
  - › intramuscular – produces peaks and troughs in pain relief and injection can be painful
  - › intravenous – the most commonly used and the dose can be titrated to effect
  - › patient-controlled analgesia (PCA) – the patient determines his or her own analgesic requirement
  - › epidural or spinal – provides good analgesia for 12–24 hours.

Morphine

- Represents the gold standard against which all analgesics are compared
- The usual dose is 5–15 mg given intravenously in small increments, titrated to response
- The peak effect is reached in 15–30 minutes, and the action lasts 3–4 hours
- Oral preparations (morphine sulphate liquid, tablets or capsules, some of which may be modified release) have half the potency of the intravenous preparation
- May also be administered via intrathecal or epidural routes (0.1–0.3 mg and up to 5 mg, respectively; higher doses result in a higher frequency of side effects)

Diamorphine

- More lipid soluble than morphine, it crosses the blood–brain barrier more rapidly (hence the 'high') and has a more rapid onset of action
- Decreases the sympathetic drive and relieves the anxiety associated with pain
- Twice as potent as morphine
- Usual intravenous dose 2.5–5 mg
- May also be administered via intrathecal (0.2–1.0 mg) or epidural routes (5 mg); higher doses result in a higher frequency of side effects

Fentanyl

- 100 times more potent than morphine
- Quicker onset (5 minutes) and shorter duration of action (45–60 minutes)
- Often used in intrathecal and epidural analgesia, either as single bolus or as part of infusion with local anaesthetics

Alfentanil

- 10 times more potent than morphine
- Very quick onset (1 minute) and short duration of action (15–30 minutes)

Codeine

- Usually administered for mild to moderate pain
- 10 times less potent than morphine
- Usual oral dose 30–60 mg 4 hourly; maximum, 240 mg per 24 hours.
- Part of its analgesic action relies on the products of its metabolism; not all individuals are able to metabolise codeine in this way, hence the variability of its effect

Dihydrocodeine

- Has a similar efficacy as codeine. However it is slightly more potent and has more of an analgesic effect independent of its metabolites
- Usual dose 30–60 mg 4 hourly; maximum 240 mg per 24 hours

Tramadol

- 5–10 times less potent than morphine
- Available in oral and injectable preparations
- Usual oral dose 50–100 mg 4 hourly; maximum 400 mg per 24 hours
- Causes less constipation and respiratory depression than morphine and other opiates

Oxycodone

- 1.5 times more potent than morphine
- Has been reported to cause fewer hallucinations, nausea and pruritis than morphine
- May be given intravenously or orally, with liquid, capsule or tablet forms available

Pethidine

- 10 times less potent than morphine
- Available in oral and injectable preparations
- Parenteral administration induces more nausea and vomiting than morphine
- Can be used to treat post-operative shivering (25 mg intravenously)

PATIENT-CONTROLLED ANALGESIA[1,2,3]

The patient is given a syringe driver with a switch that allows him or her to request repeated doses of opioid. It provides better titration of analgesic dose to pain than boluses administered by carers. The bolus dose is set so that sedation would occur before respiratory depression, acting as a safety mechanism. To prevent overdose, only the patient is allowed to press the button. No other opioids should be prescribed while on a PCA (e.g. codeine). Fluids are infused to ensure patency of the vein and a unidirectional valve should be fitted to prevent accumulation of the opioid in the giving set. Supplementary oxygen should be provided.

- Usual bolus doses are:
  > morphine: 1 mg
  > fentanyl: 20–40 mcg
  > pethidine: 10 mg
  > diamorphine: 0.5 mg
  > tramadol: 20 mg
  > oxynorm: 1 mg.
- The lock-out interval is typically 5 minutes, with no background infusion running
- Regular anti-emetics (e.g. ondansetron 4 mg 8 hourly) may help reduce the incidence of nausea
- Fentanyl may be a safer option in patients with renal impairment
- Before the PCA is commenced a good level of analgesia should be achieved using opioids boluses given by you until the patient is pain-free
- The PCA should ideally be attached to a dedicated intravenous cannula with an infusion of fluid running through the same port.

OPIOID TOXICITY

It is vital that you can recognise and treat opioid toxicity.
- Suspect it if the patient has:
  > a decreased level of consciousness
  > a decreased respiratory rate
  > small pupils.
- Treat with naloxone, usual dose 0.2–0.4 mg intravenously.

- The dose can be repeated up to a total of 10 mg. The effect lasts 30–40 minutes, so further doses may be required when long-acting opioids have been given.
- If needed, a naloxone infusion can be started. The usual hourly dose is 60% of the 'wake-up' dose.

EPIDURAL ANALGESIA[1,2,3]

Epidural analgesia can be one of the most effective forms of post-operative analgesia, but it is invasive and it has complications. It should only be considered when the anticipated pain is significant – for example, abdominal, thoracic or major orthopaedic surgery.

It can be delivered in the following ways.

- *A continuous infusion*. This is the easiest technique and requires the least intervention from nursing staff. The overall dose of local anaesthetic is higher, hence an increased risk of side effects.
- *Boluses*. These reduce the total amount given but they require staff presence, and delays in administration can result in significant pain.
- *Patient-controlled epidural analgesia*. This is the most effective technique but it requires sophisticated equipment that is not always available. Typical epidural preparations include the following:
  - > bupivacaine: (0.125% = 1.25 mg/mL)
  - > ropivacaine: (0.2% = 2 mg/mL)
  - > fentanyl: (2–4 mcg/mL) – usually an adjuvant to the local anaesthetic, as a pre-mixed solution.

The infusion rate for thoracic or lumbar epidural is 6–15 mL/hour. For patient-controlled infusion, a regimen might comprise a background infusion of 4–6 mL/hour, boluses of 2–4 mL at 10–30 minutes, up to a maximum total hourly dose of 12 mL.

If the epidural bag contains an opioid, care must be taken to avoid other opioids being given via an alternative route, as the effects may be additive and cumulative. If the epidural infusion containing an opioid is not providing sufficient pain relief, then the solution for infusion should be changed to a plain local anaesthetic one (e.g. bupivacaine 0.125%), and an opioid given via a PCA.

Epidural insertion is explained in Chapter 27.

INTRATHECAL ANALGESIA[1,3,9,10]

If an opioid is added to the local anaesthetic used for spinal anaesthesia, it can provide good analgesic cover for 18–24 hours. The adverse effects are the same as for the other routes (nausea, pruritus, respiratory depression) and they can be delayed, up to 24 hours later.

Typical doses of intrathecal opioids are:

- fentanyl: 10–25 mcg
- morphine: 100–300 mcg
- diamorphine: 100–400 mcg.

Performing spinal anaesthesia is explained in Chapter 27.

PERIPHERAL NERVE BLOCKS

Peripheral nerve blockade can provide good pain relief, minimising the use of post-operative opioids. It can be delivered as a one-off bolus, by repeated boluses or continuous infusion via a catheter.

A one-off injection can provide analgesia for up to 12 hours, depending on the agent used (*see* Table 13.1).[8]

TABLE 13.1 The concentration, maximum dose and duration of action of peripheral nerve block for different local anaesthetics (Adapted from Neill S. *Pharmacology of Regional Anaesthesia*)

Local anaesthetic	Concentration	Maximum dose	Duration (hours)
Lidocaine	1%, 2%	7 mg/kg with epinephrine (1:200 000) 3 mg/kg without epinephrine	1–4
Prilocaine	0.5%, 1%, 2%	9 mg/kg with epinephrine (1:200 000) 7 mg/kg without epinephrine	1–4
Bupivacaine	0.25%, 0.5%	2 mg/kg	3–12
Levobupivacaine	0.25%, 0.5%, 0.75%	2.5 mg/kg	3–12
Ropivacaine	0.2%, 0.75%, 1%	3 mg/kg	3–12

For perineural catheter infusions, a usual infusion rate is 5–14 mL/hour, of:
- bupivacaine: 0.1%, 0.125%
- levobupivacaine: 0.1%, 0.2%
- ropivacaine: 0.2%.

LOCAL ANAESTHETIC WOUND INFUSION

The infiltration of local anaesthetic not only provides analgesia but also appears to reduce the local inflammatory response to trauma or surgery. They can be administered in surgical wounds, intra-articularly, or instilled into cavities (e.g. the peritoneum).

REFRACTORY POST-OPERATIVE PAIN

Sometimes pain does not respond to standard therapy and requires adjuvant measures.[1] As a first step reassurance must be given, and sometimes this can help settle the pain down. If it fails, then the reason why the pain relief has failed must be sought (inadequate dose given, patchy epidural). If the patient has already had large doses of opioids (as usually is the case) then further doses might cause significant side effects. It might be that low doses of the following agents might be tried. Seek senior advice.

Midazolam

- Small intravenous doses of 0.5–1 mg might help relieve the anxiety associated with surgery and help reduce pain

Tramadol

- Works on different receptors than standard opioids

- 25–100 mg may be given intravenously
- Nausea may be a problem

Ketamine

- Ketamine is a powerful sedative that has analgesic properties
- 10–15 mg may be given intravenously
- Care must be taken with subsequent doses, not to anaesthetise the patient!
- An alternative could be oral ketamine, 10–30 mg, 6 to 8 hourly[11]
- Intra-nasal and rectal routes are also available
- Side effects include sedation, tachycardia, hypertension, nausea and hallucinations

Clonidine

- Doses of 25 mcg (up to 150 mcg) can be given
- Especially useful if the patient is hypertensive and tachycardic
- Care must be taken, as it can cause hypotension and bradycardia – wait for at least 15 minutes before giving a subsequent dose

Entonox

- Mix of 50% oxygen and 50% nitrous oxide
- Comparable with strong opioids
- Provides only very short-term pain relief (minutes)
- Should not be used if patient has an air-containing closed space, as nitrous oxide will diffuse into the space and increase the pressure (e.g. pneumothorax)

GUIDANCE FOR TREATMENT OPTIONS

The examples given in Figure 13.1 represent levels of pain commonly experienced and are subject to individual variation. Contra-indications may apply.

Key points
- The type of surgery will predict, to some degree, the amount and type of pain that will be experienced.
- Pain has an emotional component and is subjective. Use pain scores to assess pain.
- Use the analgesic ladder to build up the correct amount of analgesia.
- Be able to recognise and treat opioid toxicity.
- PCA can be used to more effectively titrate opioid doses and reduce side effects.
- Epidurals and peripheral nerve blocks have the potential to completely eradicate pain.
- Other drugs, such as sedatives, may be needed for refractory pain.

REFERENCES

1. Macintyre PE, Schug SA, Scott DA, *et al.*, editors; APM:SE Working Group of the Australian and New Zealand College of Anaesthetists and Faculty of Pain Medicine. *Acute Pain*

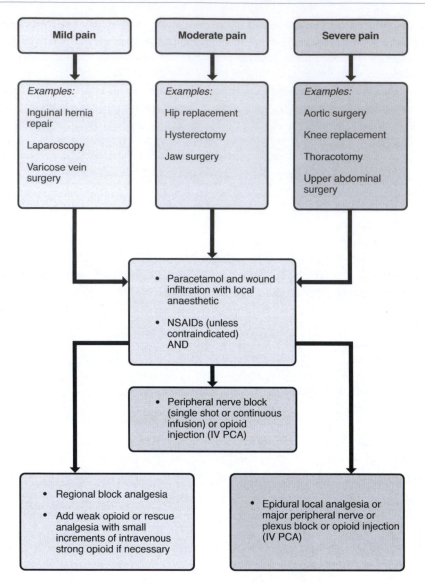

FIGURE 13.1 Predictions of pain and analgesic strategies for different types of surgery (adapted from the European Society of Regional Anaesthesia and Pain Therapy[2])

Management: scientific evidence. 3rd ed. Melbourne: ANZCA & FPM; 2010. Available at: www.anzca.edu.au/resources/books-and-publications/acutepain.pdf (accessed 10 October 2011).

2. European Society of Regional Anaesthesia and Pain Therapy. *Postoperative Pain Management – Good Clinical Practice: general recommendations and principles for successful pain management.* Available at: www.nesra.co.uk/files/acutepain/PostoperativePainManagement.pdf (accessed 10 October 2011).

3. Bonnet F (Chairman of Working Group). PROSPECT Procedure Specific Postoperative Pain Management. Available at: www.postoppain.org

4. Oxford League Table of Analgesics in Acute Pain. 2007. Available at: www.medicine.ox.ac.uk/bandolier/booth/painpag/acutrev/analgesics/leagtab.html and www.medicine.ox.ac.uk/bandolier/booth/painpag/acutrev/analgesics/lftab.html (accessed 17 October 2011).

5. *British National Formulary. No. 65.* London: BMJ Group and Pharmaceutical Press; 2013.

6. NSW Therapeutic Advisory Group. *Paracetamol Use.* (Dec 2008; with Addendum, Dec 2012). Available at: www.ciap.health.nsw.gov.au/nswtag/reviews/position-statements.html (accessed 25 April 2013.)

7. Knight SJ, von Gunten C (Co-principal Investigators). Changing Routes of Administration of Opioids. Opioid Equivalency Table. 2004. Available at: http://endoflife.northwestern.edu/pain_management/table.pdf (Hosted by The Robert H. Lurie Comprehensive Cancer Centre; funded by grant from National Cancer Institute). (accessed 10 October 2011).

8. Neill S. *Pharmacology of Regional Anaesthesia.* Available at: www.frca.co.uk/article.aspx?articleid=100816 (accessed 9 January 2012).

9. Hindle A. Intrathecal opioids in the management of acute postoperative pain. *Cont Educ Anaesth Crit Care Pain.* 2008; **8**(3): 81–5.

10. Elissa DE. Analgesic efficacy of intrathecal diamorphine for postoperative pain relief after major lumbar spine surgery. *Ain Shams J Anaesthesiol.* 2011; **4**(3): 11–20.

11. Friedman R, Jallo J, Young WF. Oral ketamine for opioid-resistant acute pain. *J Pain.* 2001; **2**(1): 75–6.

CHAPTER 14

Drugs that put you to sleep

DANIEL COTTLE

An induction agent is the start of most anaesthetics, and there are surprisingly few. Here we will discuss the intravenous induction agents. Gas inductions with inhalational anaesthetics are explained in Chapter 15. The most important to thing to remember about induction agents is that they induce anaesthesia. Obvious you might think, but once a patient is unconscious, they are likely to:

- loose control of his or her airway
- stop breathing
- become hypotensive.

These are all serious and life-threatening side effects, and you must ensure you are qualified to deal with them if you are to induce them.

The 'standard anaesthetic technique' is to induce anaesthesia with a quick-acting intravenous agent. These are mostly short-acting and provide an immediate, deep plane of anaesthesia that will allow control of the airway to take place. The patient must then be kept asleep with either an infusion of intravenous agent or volatile gas. There are advantages and disadvantages of each, which will be considered for each individual drug.

PROPOFOL
What is it?
- Propofol is the standard intravenous anaesthetic agent in the West.
- It comes in 1% and 2% preparations with an emulsion of soybean oil, glycerol and egg phosphatide, giving it the appearance of white paint. The 2% solution is reserved for infusions. Draw it up neat in a 20 mL syringe using careful antiseptic non-touch technique precautions, as it can support bacterial growth.

How does it work?
- Its mechanism of action isn't fully understood but it may prolong the action of GABA at its receptors.

How is it used?
- Inject it as a single push and warn the patient that he or she is likely to feel a

cold, or painful sensation (particularly in a small vein), but that the sensation will be gone when he or she wakes up.

- Adding 20 mg lignocaine to the syringe can reduce this effect.
- The dose of propofol varies according to other factors. The adult dose is 1.5–2.5 mg/kg.
- It causes anaesthesia in one arm-brain time (about 40 seconds). Its effects on each organ system have been summarised in Table 14.1.
- The dose needs to be increased for children and young adults, decreased for the elderly and when given with other sedatives and opioids.
- There is no need to adjust the dose for patients with hepatic or renal failure.

Pharmacokinetics

- Propofol is lipid soluble and 98% of it is protein bound in the plasma.
- Its rapid offset of action is due to redistribution to other vessel-rich organs. Its redistribution half-life (and hence the half-life to waking) is 1–2 minutes.
- It takes hours to be eliminated from the body by glucuronidation in the liver. A very small amount is eliminated in the urine and there is also an unknown metabolic pathway independent of these two.
- It has no active metabolites and causes very few allergic reactions.

TABLE 14.1 The pharmacodynamic effects of propofol

Organ system	Useful effects	Unwanted effects
Neurological	Anaesthesia and sedation	Spontaneous, jerky movements
	Reduction in cerebral metabolic rate, oxygen demand and intracranial pressure	
	Anticonvulsant	
Respiratory	Obtunds airway response to LMA	Hypoventilation or apnoea
	Prevents coughing	Loss of airway
Cardiovascular	Decreased sympathetic response	Vasodilation
		Negative inotropy causing hypotension
		Loss of baroreflex response
Others	Reduces PONV (after infusion)	Hyperlipidaemia and infusion syndrome
	Reduces intra-ocular pressure	

LMA, laryngeal mask airway; PONV, post-operative nausea and vomiting

Total intravenous anaesthesia

These properties mean that it is commonly used as an infusion for 'total intravenous anaesthesia'. This is done using specific infusion pumps that calculate the concentration of propofol in the circulation and the central nervous system. This is 'target controlled anaesthesia' and it allows you to programme a concentration of propofol in the brain with the infusion pump controlling the flow rates. Typically anaesthesia occurs at brain (or effect site) concentration of 4.0–8.0 mcg/mL, with dose adjustments the same as the induction dose. After prolonged infusion it begins to accumulate, first in muscles then fat. This prevents redistribution and prolongs the time to waking. After 2 hours, the redistribution half-life becomes 20 minutes. Target controlled anaesthesia pumps are programmed to allow for this.

Propofol infusions have been linked to paediatric deaths on intensive care and it is not licensed for infusion in children under 16 years old.

THIOPENTONE
What is it?
- This short-acting barbiturate was the anaesthetic of choice before the introduction of propofol.
- It is stored as thiopentone 500 mg, as a yellow powder and should be mixed with 20 mL of water to make 25 mg/mL.

How does it work?
- It binds to the $GABA_A$ receptor and holds it open. This then prolongs the influx of chloride into the neuron, which prevents it repolarising and so inhibits further action potentials. This neuronal inhibition causes anaesthesia.

How is it used?
- It still has some advantages over propofol, and several disadvantages. It has a slightly faster onset of action and causes less hypotension and so it's still used for a classic rapid sequence induction (RSI).
- When used for a RSI the dose is 3–7 mg/kg and the same dose adjustments should be used as for propofol. Inject as a single push.
- The effects of thiopentone on each organ system, as compared with propofol, are summarised in Table 14.2. Its properties mean that it is the drug of choice for a RSI for acute head injury, raised intracranial pressure, raised ocular pressure and status epilepticus.

Pharmacokinetics
- At the alkaline pH within this mixture the thiopentone is water-soluble. When injected into the plasma the neutral pH causes the thiopentone to become lipid-soluble, allowing it to cross the blood–brain barrier.
- It induces anaesthesia in one arm-brain time and slightly faster than propofol. After a single dose it has a similar redistribution half-life.
- It is 80% protein bound and so the dose should be reduced in patients with hypoproteinaemia, as there will be a higher proportion of active, unbound drug.
- Thiopentone is oxidised in the liver. These enzyme systems are quickly saturated, and after multiple doses the metabolism of thiopentone changes from first order to zero order kinetics. That means that the rate of metabolism is constant regardless of the serum concentration of the thiopentone and it begins to accumulate. This prolongs its duration of action considerably, and in an unpredictable way.
- This means that it isn't used as an infusion for anaesthesia.

Unwanted effects
- It precipitates with rocuronium and so the two should be separated with a saline flush.

- It can cause severe necrosis if injected intra-arterially and this should never happen.
- Thiopentone has many drug interactions. It induces the cytochrome P450 enzyme systems and so reduces the actions of other drugs.
- It also precipitates a crisis of acute intermittent porphyria. This is a rare syndrome in which certain drugs, foods and metabolic states disrupt the synthesis of the haem portion of haemoglobin and excess porphyrin production. These then go on to cause peripheral and autonomic neuropathy and coma.

TABLE 14.2 Comparing the pharmacodynamic effects of propofol and thiopentone

Organ system	Thiopentone compared with propofol
Neurological	A greater drop in cerebral metabolic rate, oxygen consumption and intracranial pressure
	Can induce an EEG burst suppression coma
	Better anticonvulsant
	No jerky movements
Respiratory	Similar dose-dependent hypoventilation and apnoea
	Less obtunding of response to LMA
Cardiovascular	Negative inotropy, less vasodilatation
	Doesn't blunt the baroreflex response
Others	Greater reduction of intra-ocular pressure
	No effect on PONV

EEG, electroencephalogram; LMA, laryngeal mask airway; PONV, post-operative nausea and vomiting

ETOMIDATE
What is it?
- Etomidate does not reduce the heart rate or systemic vascular resistance and can be used for patients in whom a drop in blood pressure is undesirable or deadly.
- There are two preparations containing etomidate 20 mg in 10 mL (2 mg/mL); one as a clear fluid and another as an emulsion, much the same as propofol.

How is it used?
- It should be drawn up and given neat at 0.3 mg/kg.
- It can be very painful on injection and the emulsion preparation reduces this. Again, lignocaine can be added to reduce pain further.
- Induction takes slightly longer than one arm-brain time and you should pause before giving the suxamethonium if etomidate is being used for an RSI.
- The dose does not need to be adjusted for elderly patients, as it does not cause hypotension.

Pharmacokinetics
- Offset of action is by redistribution in 5–7 minutes.
- It is metabolised by plasma esterases, the inactive compounds being eliminated in the urine.

Unwanted effects

- Etomidate suppresses the adrenal cortex and cortisone release. For this reason, many anaesthetists no longer use it for septic or shocked patients and those undergoing major surgery.
- Continuous infusion increases mortality in intensive care unit patients, preventing its use in this setting.
- It also causes post-operative nausea and vomiting and triggers porphyria.

MIDAZOLAM

What is it?

- It is a short-acting benzodiazepine.
- Midazolam comes prepared in an acidic, aqueous solution of varying concentrations; the safest for the anaesthetic room is 1 mg/mL. More concentrated preparations can be diluted.

How does it work?

- Like thiopentone, it also acts at the $GABA_A$ receptor, but it increases the *rate* of opening of the channel allowing a greater influx of chloride ions into the neuron.
- It is a sedative, an anxiolytic and it causes amnesia.

How is it used?

- All of the benzodiazepines will cause anaesthesia if given in large enough doses.
- Midazolam is the only one with a short enough duration of action to be realistically used as an induction agent. That said it's rarely used as an induction agent, except sometimes for cardiac surgery or shocked patients.
- More commonly it is used as an 'instant pre-med' as part of balanced anaesthesia.
- 1–2 mg at induction, along with an opioid, significantly reduces the dose of propofol or thiopentone needed.
- It produces its effects in 1–2 minutes and lasts for 30 minutes.
- Because it causes less hypotension than propofol it allows for a more cardiovascularly stable induction.
- Some anaesthetists use it to avoid patient awareness although this effect has not been proven.
- It can be used as an infusion for prolonged sedation and is the preferred agent for paediatric intensive care unit sedation.

Pharmacokinetics

- Once in the serum's pH 7.45, the midazolam changes structure and becomes lipid soluble, allowing it to cross the blood–brain barrier.
- It is metabolised in the liver with active metabolites that are excreted in the urine.
- It should be used in caution in patients with hepatic and renal failure.
- It accumulates in the tissues and its half-life increases with the length of infusion. After several days infusing (e.g. on intensive care), it can take many hours or days for the patient to wake up because it has diffused throughout the body.

Unwanted effects

- It causes dose-dependent respiratory depression and can cause airway obstruction, especially when given with opioids.
- Benzodiazepines, opioids and propofol have a synergistic relationship and even small doses of midazolam and fentanyl can cause apnoea in the elderly.
- It causes hypotension in hypovolaemic patients and lowers the blood pressure when raised.

Reversal

- Unlike the other induction agents, it is possible to reverse the actions of midazolam with *flumazanil*.
- The latter is an antagonist at the benzodiazepine GABA$_A$ receptor and can reverse benzodiazepine actions in 1–2 minutes. It only lasts for 20 minutes and an infusion should be started if longer acting benzodiazepines have been used.
- Flumazanil should only be used when there is a definite history of a pure benzodiazepine overdose, usually after administration in hospital. It may cause seizures when given after tricyclic antidepressant drugs and should never be used to reverse an unknown overdose in the emergency department.

KETAMINE

What is it?

- Ketamine is the most unusual of the induction agents. It produces a dissociative anaesthesia.
- The patient may have open eyes and appear to stare into space, while not responding to painful stimuli. What makes it even more unusual is that it raises the heart rate and blood pressure; it maintains ventilation and laryngeal reflexes and produces significant analgesia.
- It is a clear, colourless solution of ketamine 10 mg/mL. The anaesthetic dose is 10 mg/kg; for sedation use 1 mg/kg intravenously (can use repeated doses) or 10 mg/kg intramuscularly.

How does it work?

- It antagonises the excitatory action of glutamine at the NMDA receptor, producing dissociative anaesthesia.
- Its effects on each organ system are summarised in Table 14.3.

How is it used?

- It is used successfully for sedation in children (who seem to find the hallucinations less unpleasant).
- It can be used as an induction agent and in severe trauma or ruptured aortic aneurysm where the increase in blood pressure maybe life saving.
- Anaesthesia occurs in 1–2 minutes and it redistributes in 7–10 minutes.
- It can be used as an infusion and will accumulate over time (it also has active metabolites).
- It causes bronchodilatation, and infusions can be started for intubated patients with severe asthma.

Unwanted effects

- If ketamine sounds too good to be true, it is. Its use is limited because it can produce unpleasant confusion, hallucinations and delirium on emergence.
- The patient should be warned of the possibility of hallucinations or nightmares afterwards and the patient should be recovered in a quiet area.
- Ketamine should be avoided in patients with severe ischaemic heart disease, recent myocardial infarction, heart failure, head injury, intracranial tumour or haemorrhage.

TABLE 14.3 The pharmacodynamic effects of ketamine

Organ system	Effects of ketamine
Neurological	Dissociative anaesthesia, analgesia, hallucinations
	Raised intracranial pressure
	Nystagmus, jerking muscle movements, increased muscle tone
Respiratory	Maintains ventilation
Cardiovascular	Sympathetic actions increase heart rate, SVR and blood pressure
	Increase cardiac oxygen consumption
	Arrhythmias
Airway	Maintains a patent airway (but not guaranteed)
	Increased saliva secretions (can make intubation difficult)
Others	PONV
	Raised intra-ocular and uterine pressures

SVR, systemic vascular resistance; PONV, post-operative nausea and vomiting

SUMMARY

Each of the different induction agents has different properties that will make it more or less appealing in different circumstances. You will have to balance the patient factors against needs of the surgery in order to decide which to use.

Key points

- All of the induction agents cause unconsciousness and can also cause the patient to loosen his or her airway.
- Propofol is the most commonly used because of its rapid onset and offset of action. It can cause profound hypotension.
- Thiopentone provides better conditions for a rapid sequence induction.
- Midazolam, etomidate and ketamine may cause less cardiovascular collapse, but their other side effects have prevented them becoming the commonly used agents.
- Midazolam can be used alongside propofol as part of a balanced anaesthetic.

CHAPTER 15

Drugs to keep you asleep: the inhalational agents

KATE BAILEY

Inhalational anaesthetic agents are frequently used to keep patients asleep during an operation and occasionally used as induction agents in special circumstances. Unfortunately, the mechanisms by which these agents work are incompletely understood. The most commonly cited theory is the Meyer–Overton hypothesis; this suggests that inhalational agents dissolve in the lipid membranes of the neurones causing anaesthesia. The proposed evidence to support this is the link between the lipid solubility and the potency of the agents.

Ideal agents are inert, stable, non-irritant gases. They have a rapid onset and offset of action, produce minimal metabolites and side effects and provide some level of analgesia. None of the volatiles meet these criteria, so the patient, the type of surgery being performed and your own personal preference will govern the one that you choose.

MINIMUM ALVEOLAR CONCENTRATION

Minimum alveolar concentration (MAC) in simplistic terms is used to describe the potency of inhalational anaesthetic agents. It is the concentration of the agent in the alveoli required to render 50% of subjects unresponsive to a standard painful stimulus. The lower the MAC the greater the potency of the agent. Table 15.1 gives examples of factors affecting MAC.

TABLE 15.1 Factors affecting minimum alveolar concentration (MAC)

Factors affecting MAC	Increased MAC	Decreased MAC
Temperature	Pyrexia	Hypothermia
Age	Younger age	Advancing age
Thyroid function	Thyrotoxicosis	Hypothyroidism
Sympatho-adrenal stimulation	Hypercapnia	Hypocapnia, hypotension
Drugs	Chronic alcohol	Nitrous oxide, sedative drugs, acute alcohol
Other		Pregnancy

FACTORS AFFECTING THE ONSET OF INHALATIONAL AGENTS

Onset of anaesthesia, when using inhalational agents, occurs when the concentration of the agent in the alveoli reaches equilibrium with the concentration in the blood. Factors that can alter the speed with which this occurs are outlined here.

Delivering a high agent load to the alveoli

This can be achieved by using a high alveolar ventilation rate, a high inspired concentration of the agent or by utilising the second gas effect (explained shortly). High alveoli concentrations allow rapid equilibrium with the blood and a quicker onset of anaesthesia.

Cardiac output

A high cardiac output will maintain the concentration gradient between the alveoli and the blood and will consequently take a longer time to achieve steady state, thus slowing the onset of anaesthesia.

Blood:gas coefficient

Each agent has its own blood:gas coefficient. This describes how soluble an agent is in blood. *The higher the value, the greater the solubility of the agent.* The more soluble an agent is the longer it will take to reach equilibrium in the blood and thus the slower the onset of action as it is the fraction that remains insoluble that exerts a partial pressure and causes anaesthesia.

The second gas effect

The second gas effect occurs when an agent is delivered to the alveoli in a mixture of oxygen and a second carrier gas, either nitrous oxide or xenon. The effect occurs because the second carrier gas diffuses into the blood more rapidly than nitrogen can return to the alveoli, leaving a relatively increased concentration of agent in the alveoli. This increased concentration increases the gradient between the alveoli and the blood and thus increases diffusion. Consequently equilibrium is reached quicker and the speed of onset of anaesthesia is increased.

Oil:gas coefficients

Oil:gas coefficients describe an agent's solubility in lipids. Agents with high coefficients are very soluble and therefore large quantities enter the body's adipose tissue. This has consequences for the duration of action of the agent. If more of a drug is stored in fat it will take longer for it to diffuse back into the blood stream and be excreted at the end of anaesthesia, thus as a consequence the patient will take longer to wake up.

COMMONLY USED AGENTS

Sevoflurane

Sevoflurane is one of the most commonly used agents as it has many desirable properties, which make it uncomplicated, safe and efficient to use. It has a non-irritant odour and therefore it is a good agent for gas induction. Its boiling point ensures it is in the liquid state at room temperature. It has a moderately low MAC, suggesting it has high potency. Its blood:gas coefficient is quite low so is one of the more rapidly acting agents. Its oil:gas coefficient is middle of the range for the commonly used agents. Therefore, wake up is quick and predictable. Some concerns have been raised about sevoflurane's metabolites and the compounds produced when it is used in a circuit with soda lime. However, neither has been demonstrated to be renally toxic in the levels used in anaesthesia (*see* Table 15.2).

TABLE 15.2 The pharmacodynamic effects of sevoflurane

Location	Effect
Respiratory	Reduced minute ventilation, reduced respiratory drive to hypoxia, bronchodilatation
Cardiovascular	Reduced systemic vascular resistance, mild reduction in cardiac contractility, reduced blood pressure
Cerebral	Increased cerebral blood flow, raised intracranial pressure, reduced cerebral oxygen requirements
Uterus	Relaxation of the uterus

Isoflurane

Isoflurane is another commonly used agent. It has a pungent smell and is an irritant to the airways, so it is not a good agent for gas induction. It has a low MAC and a moderately low blood:gas coefficient so it has a relatively quick onset. Its oil:gas coefficient is only slightly higher than that of sevoflurane, thus recovery is a little slower. It has minimal metabolites with little risk of renal or liver toxicity (*see* Table 15.3).

TABLE 15.3 The pharmacodynamic effects of isoflurane

Location	Effect
Respiratory	Reduced minute ventilation, increased respiratory rate, airway irritability
Cardiovascular	Reduced systemic vascular resistance, mild reduction in cardiac contractility, increased heart rate, reduced blood pressure, coronary steal syndrome
Cerebral	Minimal increase in cerebral blood flow, reduced cerebral oxygen requirements
Uterus	Relaxation of the uterus

Desflurane

Desflurane is becoming increasingly popular in everyday practice. Its extremely low blood:gas coefficient and oil:gas coefficient means it has a very rapid onset and offset of action. It has minimal metabolites and has similar systemic effects to the other more commonly used agents. However, its use is slightly complicated. Its boiling point is just above room temperature and therefore, to guarantee delivered concentrations, it requires a special heated vaporiser. It is an extreme irritant to the airways and it is pungent so it cannot be used for gas induction and it can be difficult to allow patients to breathe spontaneously on it (*see* Table 15.4).

TABLE 15.4 The pharmacodynamic effects of desflurane

Location	Effect
Respiratory	Reduced minute ventilation, increased respiratory rate, airway irritability
Cardiovascular	Reduced systemic vascular resistance, large increase in heart rate and blood pressure if MAC >1
Cerebral	Increase in cerebral blood flow, raised intracranial pressure, reduced cerebral oxygen requirements
Uterus	Relaxation of the uterus

MAC, minimum alveolar concentration

Halothane

Halothane is one of the older volatile agents and is commonly used in the developing world. It has a sweet smell and relaxes the airways and is a good agent for gas induction. It has high blood:gas and oil:gas coefficients and therefore has a slow onset of action and delayed recovery from anaesthesia. Its affects on the myocardium can be troublesome and it should not be used for neuroanaesthesia. Halothane hepatitis is a type of fulminant hepatic necrosis. Its incidence is 1 in 35 000, with a higher incidence in females, the obese and after previous exposure (*see* Table 15.5).

TABLE 15.5 The pharmacodynamic effects of halothane

Location	Effect
Respiratory	Reduced minute ventilation, increased respiratory rate, bronchodilatation, reduced mucociliary function and increased secretions
Cardiovascular	Reduced systemic vascular resistance, large reduction in myocardial contractility, reduced heart rate, sensitisation to catecholamines
Cerebral	Large increase in cerebral blood flow, raised intracranial pressure, reduced cerebral oxygen requirements
Uterus	Relaxation of the uterus
Other	Reduced gastrointestinal motility, post-operative shivering

Nitrous oxide

Nitrous oxide is stored as a compressed liquid. Its MAC is greater than 100% (a theoretical number) so it isn't used for anaesthesia on its own. It is used as an adjunct to other inhalational gases. It is sweet smelling and does not irritate the airways, thus it can also aid gas induction. Its extremely low blood:gas, and oil:gas coefficients ensure it has a very rapid onset and offset of action. As described earlier, it can increase the speed of onset of other inhalational agents through the second gas effect. Using the same principle, it can cause a diffusion hypoxia at the end of anaesthesia unless supplemental oxygen is given. Nitrous oxide should be avoided in patients with raised intracranial pressure due to its significant effects on cerebral blood flow. Exposure to nitrous oxide for only a short period can cause megaloblastic changes within the bone marrow. It oxidises cobalt which inhibits the enzyme methionine synthetase, reducing DNA synthesis. When blood containing nitrous oxide equilibrates with closed air spaces within the body, the volume of nitrous oxide entering will exceed that of nitrogen leaving. In expandable compartments such as the bowel this causes distension; however, in fixed compartments such as the middle ear and eye there is an increase in pressure. It should be avoided for surgery in these areas (*see* Table 15.6).

Nitrous oxide has analgesic properties that are well utilised in Entonox. This is a 50:50 mixture of nitrous oxide and oxygen. Women in labour and patients undergoing short painful procedures frequently use it. The mixture is stored as a gas but it separates into its two parts if the temperature falls below −7°C, its pseudocritical temperature. This renders the gas ineffective as an analgesic initially, as only oxygen is delivered, but dangerous as the cylinder empties and a hypoxic delivery of nitrous oxide alone occurs.

TABLE 15.6 The pharmacodynamic effects of nitrous oxide

Location	Effect
Respiratory	Minute ventilation is unchanged, diffusion hypoxia
Cardiovascular	Mild reduction in cardiac contractility, mild increase in heart rate
Cerebral	Increased cerebral blood flow, raised intracranial pressure, analgesia
Uterus	Relaxation of the uterus
Other	Post-operative nausea and vomiting, altered DNA synthesis, expansion of gases in enclosed spaces

Xenon

Xenon has been described as being extremely close to the ideal anaesthetic agent. It is an inert non-irritant gas. It has a rapid onset and offset of action, has no metabolites, is an analgesic and is cardiovascularly stable. However, xenon is extremely expensive to produce and as a result has not entered routine practice (*see* Table 15.7).

TABLE 15.7 The pharmacodynamic effects of xenon

Location	Effect
Respiratory	Minute ventilation maintained, decreased respiratory rate, increased tidal volume
Cardiovascular	Cardiovascular stability
Cerebral	Increased cerebral blood flow, raised intracranial pressure, analgesia

TABLE 15.8 A summary of the properties of volatile agents

Property	Sevoflurane	Isoflurane	Desflurane	Halothane	Nitrous oxide	Xenon
MAC	1.8%	1.15%	6.6%	0.75%	105%	71%
Blood:gas coefficient	0.7	1.4	0.45	2.5	0.47	0.14
Oil:gas coefficient	80	98	29	224	1.4	20
Metabolites	5%	0.2%	0.02%	20%	0.01%	0%

MAC, minimum alveolar concentration

GAS INDUCTION

Using inhalational agents to induce anaesthesia is desirable in two main circumstances:
1. in paediatric anaesthesia where intravenous access is not possible or practical
2. when a difficult airway has been predicted and the patient is not at increased risk of aspiration.

High concentrations are delivered to the patient by a face mask that will slowly induce anaesthesia while keeping the patient spontaneously breathing. For successful gas induction the agent selected must not irritate the airways and must have a pleasant odour. Commonly used agents are sevoflurane and halothane.

Key points

- Agents with low blood:gas coefficients act rapidly.
- Agents with low oil:gas coefficients wear off quickly.
- Desflurane requires a special vaporiser because of its low boiling point.
- Halothane sensitises the myocardium to catecholamines and can cause hepatitis.
- Nitrous oxide is a good analgesic and increases the speed of onset and reduces the MAC of other agents.
- Gas inductions must be performed with non-irritant agents.

FURTHER READING

- Peck TE, Hill SA. *Pharmacology for Anaesthesia and Intensive Care*. 3rd ed. New York: Cambridge University Press; 2004.
- Aitkenhead AR, Rowbotham DJ, Smith G. *Textbook of Anaesthesia*. 5th ed. London: Churchill Livingstone; 2007.

CHAPTER 16

Muscle relaxants

PETER FRANK AND CRAIG SPENCER

INTRODUCTION

One day, an orthopaedic surgical trainee turned to me and asked, 'When you give a muscle relaxant why doesn't the heart stop?' This is a great question, and to answer it fully you need to have an understanding of the physiology of the neuromuscular junction and how these agents block the chemical transmission that occurs there. Also, how the heart operates under its own rhythmicity, and is modulated by the autonomic rather than the somatic nervous system.

The term 'muscle relaxant' is slightly misleading and may conjure up the impression that these agents are in some way interfering with the intrinsic mechanism of muscular contraction, which they do not. Direct stimulation of a muscle belly with diathermy, for example, will cause some localised contraction despite complete inhibition of voluntary skeletal muscle contraction. Neuromuscular blocking drugs – as we shall now call them – are very specific to anaesthesia, and therefore it is unlikely you will be familiar with their use, unless you are an anaesthetist or intensivist. In this chapter we will not explore the minutiae of these agents but provide you with a practical approach to their use.

THE NEUROMUSCULAR JUNCTION

More in-depth analysis of the neuromuscular junction (NMJ) can be found in any good physiology book, but we will have a short recap here, as it is useful to keep it in mind when considering how neuromuscular blocking drugs work.

The NMJ is the junction between the terminal button of a motor neurone and the muscle fibre it innervates. The myelinated motor neuron looses its myelin sheath and forms a terminal button. This invaginates into the muscle fibre but lies outside the muscle fibre plasma membrane, separated from it by the synaptic space, which is filled with extracellular fluid. It is into this space that acetylcholine (ACh) is released when the nerve is stimulated. The binding of ACh to nicotinic ACh receptors on the post-synaptic muscle membrane leads to ion influx resulting in a muscle end-plate potential. If the signal is large enough, depolarisation of the muscle membrane occurs, causing an action potential to propagate along the muscle fibre, which in turn results in muscle contraction.

TYPES OF NEUROMUSCULAR BLOCKING DRUGS AND THEIR REVERSAL

They are divided into two main types, depolarising and non-depolarising, which refers to the effect the agent has on the post-synaptic membrane.

Depolarising relaxants

Suxamethonium is the only depolarising neuromuscular blocking drug in routine use. Structurally it is two ACh molecules joined together through their acetyl groups and therefore it mimics the action of ACh. It opens the nicotinic channels resulting in the flow of ions across the cell membrane resulting in localised membrane depolarisation. Clinically this causes muscle twitching or 'fasciculation', which usually take between 30 and 60 seconds to cease. This corresponds to the duration of onset of complete paralysis. Once the motor end plate is fully depolarised it cannot initiate any further action potentials along the muscle fibre, regardless of the amount of ACh released into the synaptic cleft.

Non-depolarising relaxants

There are several different non-depolarising neuromuscular blocking drugs with slightly different properties. However, they share the same mechanism of action, competitive binding to the alpha subunit of the nicotinic ACh receptor on the post-synaptic membrane. This means they prevent the ACh released from the nerve terminal occupying both binding sites on the nicotinic receptor and thus prevent channel opening. More than 70% of receptors need to be blocked before the effects can be observed clinically because of the excess of ACh receptors on the post-synaptic membrane.

Reversal of paralysis

- Suxamethonium is rapidly broken down by plasma cholinesterase resulting in a very short period of skeletal muscle paralysis. Some patients possess defective plasma cholinesterase resulting in a prolonged effect from suxamethonium. This rare condition is known as suxamethonium apnoea. Several autosomal recessive genes have been identified which, if present can result in paralysis lasting up to 4 hours after a single dose.
- Non-depolarising neuromuscular blocking drugs diffuse down their concentration gradient away from the NMJ and into the plasma. The rate of recovery is thus dependent on the rate of clearance from the plasma. Recovery can be expedited by giving an acetylcholinesterase inhibitor such as neostigmine. Neostigmine prevents ACh breakdown, increasing its concentration at the NMJ to a level where it can out-compete the neuromuscular blocker displacing it from its binding site and allowing normal neuromuscular transmission to resume.
- Sugammadex is a new agent, developed specifically to reverse the effects of the non-depolarising drug, rocuronium. The molecule resembles a ring doughnut in shape, the centre of which strongly binds rocuronium, preventing its action at the NMJ. Having a potent reversal agent for rocuronium is useful in emergency situations where the anaesthetist wants the patient to resume spontaneous breathing as quickly as possible.

MONITORING NEUROMUSCULAR BLOCKADE

Being able to monitor the degree of paralysis is vital when using neuromuscular blocking agents. There are several different methods used to measure neuromuscular blockade but by far the most common is visual observation of the response produced by electrical stimulation using a nerve stimulator.

Commonly used sites for attachment of the nerve stimulator electrodes include the ulnar, facial and accessory nerves. There are four main patterns of stimulation:

1. *Single twitch*. This can be used as a reference prior to blockade but it is not very useful in isolation.
2. *Train-of-four* (TOF). Four electrical pulses are administered. The TOF count is the number of palpable muscle twitches, whereas the TOF ratio is the ratio of the magnitude of the first and last twitches, sometimes also described as 'fade'. A count of three to four twitches is required before reversing the blockade can be considered. If reversal is attempted when the block is more profound, then there is a chance the reversal agent could wear off before the blockade, resulting in paralysis returning in an awake, non-anaesthetised patient.
3. *Double burst stimulation* (DBS). Two short rapid bursts of stimulation are delivered 750 ms apart. DBS is more sensitive at detecting small amounts of fade and may therefore help to ensure that a patient is fully reversed prior to waking them up.
4. *Post-tetanic count* (PTC). A 5-second tetanic stimulation at 50 Hz potentiates subsequent twitches. This allows intense neuromuscular blockade to be assessed, which would produce no twitches on TOF. The number of twitches produced following tetany gives the PTC. A PTC of 10 approximately correlates with the return of a single twitch on TOF.

EXAMPLES OF FREQUENTLY USED AGENTS

Suxamethonium

Uses

- To achieve rapid muscle relaxation during rapid sequence induction
- In the treatment of severe or life-threatening laryngospasm
- To achieve relaxation during short surgical procedures

Dose

- 0.5–1.5 mg/kg (usually 1 mg/kg of actual body weight) intravenously
- May be given intramuscularly at a dose of up to 2.5 mg/kg for adults and 4 mg/kg for children

Side effects

- Arrhythmias, most commonly bradycardia
- Hyperkalaemia due to K^+ efflux during depolarisation
- Myalgia – most common in young females who mobilise soon after exposure
- A rise in intra-ocular pressure – caution in penetrating eye injury
- Anaphylaxis
- Malignant hyperthermia, a rare autosomal-dominant disorder resulting in massive and generalised muscle contraction (treatment involves aggressive

cooling and the administration of intravenous dantrolene, which interferes with the release of calcium from the sarcoplasmic reticulum)
- Suxamethonium apnoea

Metabolism
- Rapidly broken down by plasma cholinesterase to choline and succinylmonocholine

Atracurium
Uses
- Provides intubating conditions within 90–120 seconds post intravenous administration
- May be given as an intravenous infusion to provide continual paralysis in the intensive care environment.

Dose
- 0.5 mg/kg intravenously

Side effects
- May precipitate histamine release

Metabolism
- 60% of atracurium's breakdown is by non-specific esterases which are not related to the plasma cholinesterase responsible for suxamethonium breakdown.
- Spontaneous breakdown also occurs – this is known as Hofmann elimination and occurs when atracurium is exposed to body temperature and pH (hypothermia and acidosis will slow the process – often used in renal and hepatic failure for these reasons).

Rocuronium
Uses
- Can provide rapid intubating conditions and therefore has a role in a 'modified' rapid sequence induction. The drug is relatively non-potent and therefore a large amount is required. The large quantity results in a large concentration gradient between the plasma and the NMJ, resulting in a fast onset of action.

Dose
- 0.6 mg/kg intravenously produces intubating conditions in 100–120 seconds; however, a larger dose can be used (0.9–1.2 mg/kg), which produces intubating conditions in 60 seconds

Side effects
- Minimal cardiovascular effects and less histamine release than atracurium.

Metabolism
- Rocuronium is primarily excreted in bile and therefore may accumulate in hepatic failure
- It is effectively reversed by sugammadex

Vecuronium

Uses

- Provides intubation conditions in 90–120 seconds after administration

Dose

- 0.1 mg/kg intravenously – presented as 10 mg freeze-dried powder requiring reconstitution with 5 mL water prior to administration (time-consuming to draw up, but also quite portable, as a fridge is not required)

Side effects

- Minimal cardiovascular effects and less prone to cause histamine release than atracurium. It is sometimes used in asthma for this reason

Metabolism

- Broken down in the liver with the metabolites being rapidly cleared by the kidney

Mivacurium

Uses

- It provides intubating conditions in 90–120 seconds after administration – useful for short procedures because of its rapid offset

Dose

- 0.07–0.25 mg/kg results in paralysis for 10–20 minutes

Side effects

- It can cause histamine release if given rapidly

Metabolism

- It is broken down by plasma cholinesterase into highly water-soluble metabolites – therefore patients with plasma cholinesterase deficiency are susceptible to prolonged blockade

---

Key points

- Despite being very specialised agents, neuromuscular blocking agents can be easily understood because of their simple mechanism of action.
- They are classified into depolarising and non-depolarising relaxants.
- The only depolarising agent in current use is suxamethonium, and this is used when a fast onset and offset is required (i.e. during a rapid sequence induction).
- There are several different non-depolarising neuromuscular blocking agents that, despite having the same mechanism of action, vary in their speeds of onset, offset and metabolism.
- The depth of neuromuscular blockade can be assessed using a nerve stimulator. This uses four main patterns of stimulation: (1) single twitch, (2) train-of-four, (3) double burst and (4) post-tetanic count.

CHAPTER 17

Drugs that stop you vomiting

NICOLA SMITH AND KENNETH McGRATTAN

INTRODUCTION

Post-operative nausea and vomiting (PONV) is a common side effect following anaesthesia. It can be very upsetting for patients and in severe cases may cause more distress than post-operative pain. As well as being unpleasant for the patient, PONV can cause significant morbidity. Vomiting is associated with increased intracranial and intraocular pressure, and it can contribute to wound dehiscence, incisional hernias and aspiration of gastric contents into the lungs. If prolonged, PONV can cause electrolyte imbalances and dehydration. It can also lead to prolonged hospital stays – an increasingly important consideration given the financial implications and pressures on hospital beds. For these reasons, you must take great care to assess your patient's risk of PONV and minimise its occurrence.

PHYSIOLOGY OF NAUSEA AND VOMITING (EMESIS)

Nausea is defined as an unpleasant sensory experience with the urge to expel gastric contents via the vomiting reflex but it may be present without the physical act of vomiting. The vomiting reflex is a complex, protective mechanism designed to avoid ingestion of toxic substances. The reflex is coordinated by the vomiting centre located in the dorsolateral reticular formation of the medulla oblongata. Stimuli for nausea and vomiting come from many sources including the gastrointestinal tract, the chemoreceptor trigger zone, the vestibular system and higher centres of the brain. Afferent input into the vomiting centre is via the glossopharyngeal and vagus nerve from the pharynx, upper oesophagus and stomach. The vomiting centre coordinates incoming signals and brings about vomiting via the cranial and spinal nerves that supply the upper gastrointestinal tract, diaphragm and abdominal muscles.

The chemoreceptor trigger zone located near to the area postrema of the floor of the fourth ventricles bilaterally receives chemical signals from the cerebrospinal fluid and directly from the bloodstream. Therefore, it is susceptible to circulating drugs, even those that do not cross the blood–brain barrier. Neurotransmitters thought to be involved in this region include acetylcholine, serotonin, histamine, dopamine and substance P.

RISK FACTORS FOR PONV

Anaesthetists assess individual patients at the preoperative visit and make a note of factors that might increase their risk of PONV. Broadly categorised, these risks can be grouped into patient factors, surgical factors and anaesthetic factors.

Patient factors increasing the risk of PONV

- Female gender
- History of PONV or motion sickness
- Children
- Non-smokers

Surgical factors increasing the risk of PONV

- Ear, nose and throat, abdominal, gynaecological, and squint surgery
- Preoperative dehydration

Anaesthetic factors increasing the risk of PONV

- Use of nitrous oxide
- Gastric insufflation (during bag or mask ventilation)
- Use of opioid analgesia

PREVENTION OF PONV

Anaesthetists like to anticipate problems rather than react to them and so prophylaxis of emesis is favoured and has been shown to be effective in those at risk. Modifying risk factors is another strategy commonly employed by anaesthetists to minimise the risk of PONV. Patient and surgical factors are a consideration when assessing risk of PONV but cannot be modified; however, anaesthetic factors can often be tailored accordingly. Regional blocks and local anaesthetic may be considered appropriate to avoid a general anaesthetic altogether. If a general anaesthetic is necessary, shorter-acting anaesthetic agents (e.g. propofol, remifentanil) are generally felt to be beneficial. Avoiding nitrous oxide and overuse of bag and mask ventilation at induction of anaesthesia may also help to prevent sickness after general anaesthetic.

Apfel *et al.*[1] devised a simple scoring system used to assess risk of PONV. One point was given for each of the following four risk factors:

1. female gender
2. non-smoker
3. past history of PONV or motion sickness
4. use of post-operative opioids.

A score of 0, 1, 2, 3 or 4 gave an approximate PONV risk of 10%, 20%, 40%, 60% and 80%, respectively. This simple-to-remember and easily applicable scoring system is an approach to guide use of prophylactic anti-emetics during general anaesthesia. In practice, anaesthetists use a combination of scoring risk factors, previous experience and an individualised patient assessment to guide their practice.

PROPHYLAXIS AND TREATMENT OF PONV

Broadly grouped by their mechanism of action, there are four main categories of anti-emetics commonly used by anaesthetists:

- antihistamines
- anti-muscarinics
- serotonin antagonists
- dopamine antagonists.

Using a combination of these agents to prevent and treat PONV is an effective approach in those at high risk.

ANTI-MUSCARINICS

Examples:
- atropine
- hyoscine.

Actions:
- block acetylcholine receptors.

Side effects:
- dry mouth
- blurred vision
- urinary retention
- sedation.

The anti-muscarinics are the oldest class of anti-emetic but were initially used in anaesthesia to block the vagal side effects of chloroform and to dry secretions. They were found to be a useful anti-emetic, particularly for vestibular nerve-induced nausea and vomiting, but newer agents with fewer side effects have largely superseded them.

ANTIHISTAMINES

Examples:
- cyclizine
- promethazine.

Actions:
- antagonise histamine (H_1) receptors.

Side effects:
- sedation
- anticholinergic side effects (as mentioned earlier)
- rarely, hypotension, tachyarrhythmias, extra-pyramidal side effects and the exacerbation of closed-angle glaucoma.

Because of the tendency of cyclizine to cause tachycardia and potentially tachyarrhythmias, it is safest to administer a slow intravenous dose with electrocardiograph monitoring. Antihistamines should be avoided in severe liver disease.

SEROTONIN ANTAGONISTS

Examples:
- ondansetron
- granisetron.

Actions:
- antagonise serotonin ($5-HT_3$) receptors centrally (at the chemoreceptor trigger zone) and peripherally.

Side effects:
- headache.

Serotonin antagonists are a popular choice of anti-emetic, both as a prophylaxis and as a treatment of PONV. They work quickly, particularly when administered intravenously, and they have relatively few side effects.

DOPAMINE ANTAGONISTS

Examples:
- domperidone
- metoclopramide.

Actions:
- antagonise dopamine (D_2) receptors
- metoclopramide also acts as a prokinetic leading to increased gastric emptying.

Side effects:
- extra-pyramidal effects
- oculogyric crisis.

Metoclopramide is thought to have little efficacy for use in PONV and is not routinely administered for perioperative purposes. It should be avoided in the young, particularly girls and young females who are more susceptible to the dystonic effects.

Dexamethasone is a corticosteroid widely used by anaesthetists as an anti-emetic but the mechanism for its anti-emetic properties is not well understood. Its anti-inflammatory effects may be of additional benefit when used perioperatively but should be avoided if severe infective processes are present, as it may reduce the physiological immune response.

Key points
- PONV is a common complication of general anaesthesia and one that is feared by patients.
- Anaesthetists assess and attempt to modify identified risk factors for PONV.
- Administering appropriate anti-emetic prophylaxis can effectively reduce the incidence of PONV and need for rescue anti-emetics.
- Multimodal agents used in combination are beneficial in high-risk cases.

REFERENCE

1. Apfel CC, Läärä E, Koivuranta M, *et al*. A simplified risk score for predicting postoperative nausea and vomiting: conclusions from cross-validations between two centers. *Anesthesiology.* 1999; **91**(3): 693–700.

CHAPTER 18

Emergency drugs

JESS BRIGGS AND CLAIRE MOORE

It is vital to familiarise yourself with a list of emergency drugs. Emergencies happen frequently in anaesthesia. Feeling comfortable with a range of drugs will allow you to manipulate abnormal physiology and manage emergencies rapidly.

There are many categories of emergency drugs – some you will be required to draw up at the start of each list, while others will be kept in the drugs cupboard and drawn up when required. We recommend that the following drugs are drawn up and kept ready:

- metaraminol
- ephedrine
- atropine plus or minus glycopyrrolate
- suxamethonium (*see* Chapter 16).

FIRST, A REVIEW OF BASIC PHYSIOLOGY

Several factors combine to control the heart rate (HR), blood pressure (BP) and cardiac output (CO).

Cardiac output (CO) = stroke volume (SV) × heart rate (HR)

- Stroke volume is dependent on preload (optimal filling of the heart), contractility and afterload (force against which the heart has to pump to eject blood).
- A fluid challenge will increase venous return to the heart (preload) and increase the stroke volume.
- The force of contractility can be increased with a positively inotropic drug (via β_1 cardiac adrenoceptors or by the independent increase of calcium in the cardiac cells).
- Reducing the afterload may help a failing heart but it is likely to reduce the BP.
- The HR can be increased with a positively chronotropic drug (again via β_1 cardiac adrenoceptors). Initially increasing the HR will increase the CO but as the rate increases, the diastolic filling time reduces and a very high HR reduces the CO.

Blood pressure (BP) = cardiac output (CO) × systemic vascular resistance (SVR)

- BP is a product of the CO and the resistance provided by the vascular system (SVR). The vascular system is made of three components:
  › the arterial system provides the main resistance to CO, determines the flow to the organs and tissues, and allows the determination of a BP
  › the capillaries, although small in calibre, offer a large volume of low-pressure vessels that feed individual organs and tissues; the flow through the capillaries is directly dependent on the filling from the arterial system
  › the veins act as capacitance vessels and the blood within them forms a reservoir; increasing the venous return to the heart increases the preload and thus the CO.
- Increasing SVR can be achieved by direct stimulation of α_1 adrenoceptors causing vasoconstriction.
- In practice most drugs have effects on several receptors and thus a drug designed to increase CO may cause a reduction in BP. For example, dobutamine causes an increase in CO but a reduction in SVR – the effect on BP is variable.

THE CONCEPT OF FLOW

While we measure BP, a more physiological target is the blood flow through an organ. Ideally, this is what we should be aiming to optimise, although unlike BP, there is no easy way to directly measure flow. Targeting specific BPs can be detrimental; increasing SVR can result in reduced flow to vital organs and a reduction in CO. However, ensuring an adequate mean arterial pressure (and sufficient diastolic pressure) is necessary to give a 'driving force' through pressure dependent organs (e.g. the kidney).

Indirect measurements of adequate flow such as capillary refill time, urine output, lactate level and, if appropriate, level of consciousness can be monitored during anaesthesia.

RECEPTORS AND THE AUTONOMIC NERVOUS SYSTEM

You must understand the sympathetic and parasympathetic systems in order to appreciate the effects of drugs acting at the various receptors. Figure 18.1 shows a schematic representation of the various receptors and their functions within each system. Both systems have preganglionic and postganglionic fibres. Preganglionic fibres in both the sympathetic and parasympathetic systems synapse on ganglia releasing acetylcholine onto nicotinic receptors. The postganglionic fibres of each system however have very different effects.

The sympathetic nervous system is responsible for the 'fight or flight' reaction: it prepares the body for emergency situations by increasing CO, reducing airway resistance, and directing blood to the muscles and vital organs, and away from the skin and gut. Postganglionic fibres release noradrenaline that has actions on various adrenoceptors (α, β_1, β_2), each with different actions (*see* Table 18.1). Some sympathetic preganglionic fibres synapse straight onto the adrenal gland, releasing adrenaline, which stimulates adrenoceptors directly.

The parasympathetic nervous system often opposes the sympathetic system.

Postganglionic fibres release acetylcholine, which affects parasympathetic muscarinic receptors (of subtypes M1–3) (*see* Figure 18.1).

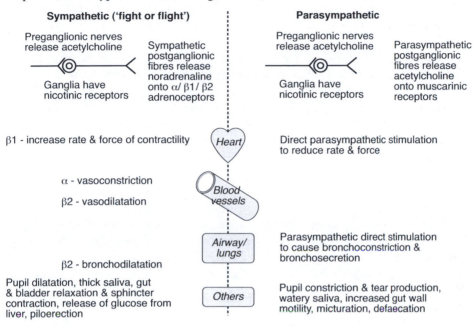

FIGURE 18.1 Sympathetic and parasympathetic nervous systems and receptors

TABLE 18.1 Adrenoceptor functions

	Useful effects	Common problems
Alpha-1 (α_1)	Vasoconstriction causing increased SVR and BP	Reduced blood flow to splanchnic, renal and coronary vasculature
Beta-1 (β_1)	Increased contractility and HR giving increased CO	Some drugs can increase myocardial work and oxygen consumption leading to ischaemia
Beta-2 (β_2)	Vasodilatation especially splanchnic and renal vasculature	Leads to reduced SVR – effect on BP depends on other properties of the drug
Dopamine receptor	Vasodilatation and diuresis	Dopamine receptors in splanchnic and renal vasculature

SVR, systemic vascular resistance; BP, blood pressure; HR, heart rate; CO, cardiac output

DRUGS USED PRIMARILY TO INCREASE THE BLOOD PRESSURE

Metaraminol

Metaraminol acts mainly by α_1 vasoconstriction, leading to an increased SVR and thus a rise in BP.

- There is an associated reflex bradycardia and transient reduction in CO.
- It also has indirect effects to increase BP and coronary blood flow, and mild but much less clinically relevant β effects.
- It is most useful for situations where there is vasodilatation (e.g. regional

anaesthesia) or where tachycardia and hypotension exist (to be given in combination with a fluid challenge).
- Because of its indirect effects, a reaction with monoamine oxidase inhibitors (MAOIs) can cause a hypertensive crisis.

Metaraminol is a very potent drug and must be diluted and used with care.
- Vials contain 10 mg in 1 mL. Dilute into 20 mL of normal saline to make a concentration of 0.5 mg/mL.
- Bolus doses of 0.2–0.5 mg (0.5–1 mL) can be used to increase BP – start with low doses, some patients are very sensitive to even a small bolus. Action is within 1–2 minutes; you will usually see the HR reduce initially.
- Metaraminol can be used by infusion (10 mg in 50 mL of normal saline) and the dose titrated to the patient's BP.

Phenylephrine

Phenylephrine is a pure direct-acting α_1 vasoconstrictor with similar properties to metaraminol. It is presented in 10 mg vials and given at a dose of 20–100 mcg bolus or as an infusion.
- Dilute 10 mg into 100 mL of saline, which can then be given as 0.5–1 mL bolus (50–100 mcg) or infused at 10–30 mL/hour.
- It does not cause reactions with MAOIs.

Ephedrine

Ephedrine has direct α and β actions at adrenoceptors and an indirect action to increase noradrenaline release from nerve terminals.
- Peripheral vasoconstriction occurs via α_1 agonism and its indirect effects increase SVR and BP.
- β_1 actions include positive inotropy and chronotropy to increase CO and HR but also myocardial work and oxygen consumption. Coronary blood flow is increased and it is a potent bronchodilator.
- It is used to *increase BP and CO* during general and regional anaesthesia and is often thought of as a more physiological agent because of its increase in CO as well as BP.
- The elevation in HR is temporary but it is a useful drug when there is already a bradycardia.
- Because of its effects on the heart it can cause dysrhythmias and its indirect effects lead to a hypertensive crisis with MAOIs. Other side effects include splanchnic and renal vasoconstriction and an amphetamine-like reaction from central stimulation.
- Repeated boluses lead to tachyphylaxis as noradrenaline stores become depleted in nerve terminals.
- It is generally more forgiving than metaraminol.

Dilution

- Vials contain 30 mg in 1 mL – dilute this into 10 mL of normal saline to make a concentration of 3 mg/mL.
- Give a 3–6 mg bolus (1–2 mL) according to response. Again, start slow – effects

can be marked and take 1–2 minutes to occur, so it is easy to give too much. You generally see an increased HR just before the increase in BP.

Noradrenaline (norepinephrine)

Noradrenaline (norepinephrine) is a far more potent drug and must be given centrally to avoid tissue necrosis.

- Its main actions are potent α_1-mediated vasoconstriction to increase SVR and BP and give a reflex bradycardia. It has much weaker β_1 effects with slightly increased contractility. Overall CO generally falls.
- It increases myocardial work; arrhythmias are rare but can result.
- Its main uses are in hypotensive states due to vasodilatation (low SVR) – e.g. sepsis and intra-operative vasodilatation. It is very short acting and therefore must be given as an infusion.
- Intense vasoconstriction can lead to ischaemic gut and reduced hepatic, renal & muscle blood flow. If used correctly the reduction in renal blood flow is usually offset by an increase in perfusion pressure to maintain or improve urine output. With prolonged use it can lead to ischaemia of the peripheries and gangrene.
- Noradrenaline alone does not perfuse organs and one must ensure that the patient is adequately fluid resuscitated before commencing a noradrenaline infusion.
- Direct arterial BP measurement via an arterial line is essential so the dose can be titrated to response.

Dilution

- Vials contain 4 mg in 4 mL (1 mg/mL) and are usually made up to 40 or 50 mL with dextrose.
- 'Single strength' noradrenaline is 4 mg made up to 40 mL (i.e. with 36 mL of dextrose). This gives a solution of 100 mcg/mL. It is usually started at 5 mL/hour.
- If large doses are required more concentrated solutions can be drawn up.
- Once commenced via a central line, there will be a delay in action due to the dead space in the infusion line. If severely hypotensive use a bolus of metaraminol or ephedrine to maintain BP. Noradrenaline should not be bolused, but the infusion rate can be cautiously increased until BP is restored (watch the arterial line and reduce the rate once BP begins to climb).

DRUGS THAT INCREASE CARDIAC CONTRACTILITY (INOTROPES)

All of the following inotropes must be given centrally with direct BP measurement via an arterial line and ideally with some form of CO monitoring to titrate response.

Adrenaline (epinephrine)

Adrenaline (epinephrine) is an extremely potent, direct acting, α and β agonist. Initially β effects predominate with increased contractility: the systolic BP normally increases, although the diastolic may fall due to β_2-induced vasodilatation. As the dose rises, there is an increase in α-mediated vasoconstriction and the BP may rise dramatically.

- Additional effects include tachycardia, bronchodilatation, increased glucose levels from insulin inhibition as well as gluconeogenesis, increase in basal metabolic rate and a reduction in gastrointestinal transit and blood flow.

TABLE 18.2 A comparison of the effects of metaraminol, ephedrine, phenylephrine and noradrenaline

	Metaraminol	Ephedrine	Phenylephrine	Noradrenaline
Action	Direct and indirect α_1 agonist Mild β action	Direct and indirect α_1 and β_1 agonist	Direct-acting α_1 agonist	Potent direct α_1 agonist Mild β_1 agonist
Predominant effects	Increased BP via vasoconstriction and increased SVR	Increased SVR and BP with increased CO and HR	Increased SVR and BP	↑SVR and BP (α_1) Mild positive inotropy (β_1)
Other actions	Reflex bradycardia, ↓CO, ↑PVR, ↑coronary blood flow (indirect mechanism)	↑Myocardial work and O_2 consumption, ↑PVR	Reflex bradycardia and slight CO reduction	Reflex bradycardia Overall CO↓ or static ↑Cerebral and coronary blood flow ↑PVR
Indications	Hypotension (especially with ↑HRs)	Hypotension (especially with ↓CO or ↓HR)	Hypotension (especially in maternity)	Hypotension from vasodilatation (e.g. sepsis)
Dose and dilution	Dilute vial (10 mg in 1 mL) into 20 mL normal saline to give 0.5 mg/mL. Bolus: 0.2–0.5 mg (0.5–1 mL). Infusion: 10 mg vial diluted into 50 mL; run at 1–10 mL/hour	Dilute vial (30 mg in 1 mL) into 10 mL saline to give 3 mg/mL. Bolus: 3–6 mg (1–2 mL)	Dilute vial (10 mg in 1 mL) into 100 mL (100 mcg/mL). Bolus: 0.2–1 mL (20–100 mcg). Infuse at 10–30 mL/hour	'Single strength': 4 mg in 40 mL dextrose. Run as infusion at 1–15 mL/hour (start at 5 mL/hour). 'Double strength': 8 mg in 40 mL
Can be given . . .	Peripherally or centrally	Peripherally or centrally	Peripherally or centrally	Centrally only

	Metaraminol	Ephedrine	Phenylephrine	Noradrenaline
Pharmacokinetics	Little known Onset in 1 minute, can last up to an hour (usually less)	Hepatic metabolism (oxidation) Resistant to monoamine oxidase and thus lasts longer than most agents 85%–99% of the unchanged drug is excreted renally Onset in 1–3 minutes, lasts up to 1 hour	Hepatic metabolism (oxidation – MAOIs) Onset in 1–2 minutes, lasts 5–10 minutes	Hepatic metabolism (by monoamine oxidases) and in the cytoplasm Renal excretion Very short half-life (0.5–2.4 minutes), must be given as an infusion
Unwanted effects	Brief ↓CO, ↓HR and ↓cerebral and renal perfusion Splanchnic vasoconstriction Large increase in BP can cause left ventricular failure and cardiac arrest Other side effects: headache, nausea, dizziness, hyperglycaemia	Central stimulation with insomnia, anxiety, chest pains and nausea Dysrhythmias Splanchnic and renal vasoconstriction Tachyphylaxis with repeated boluses	Brief reduction in CO, HR and renal perfusion Less detrimental to foetus; therefore, used in obstetrics Exaggerated response with MAOIs/TCAs	Splanchnic, renal and hepatic ischaemia Ischaemic peripheries, especially if hypovolaemic Headache, anxiety and chest pains Exaggerated response with MAOIs/TCAs
Caution	Elderly very sensitive Do not use with MAOIs/TCAs	Elderly, cardiac disease Do not use with MAOIs/TCAs	Elderly and CVS disease	Elderly, hypovolaemia

BP, blood pressure; SVR, systemic vascular resistance; CO, cardiac output; HR, heart rate; PVR, peripheral vascular resistance; MAOI, monoamine oxidase inhibitor; TCA, tricyclic antidepressant; CVS, cardiovascular system.

- Side effects include arrhythmias, myocardial ischaemia and cerebral haemorrhage from massive rises in BP. Splanchnic and peripheral vasoconstriction may be problematic. Again, ensure the patient is adequately fluid resuscitated.

Dilution

- 1 mL vial of 1:1000 = 1 mg in 1 mL.
- 10 mL vial of 1:10 000 = 1 mg in 10 mL (100 mcg/mL).
- Found in pre-packed mini-jets.
- In peri-arrest situations and hypotension, adrenaline may be used in a very dilute form when other drugs have failed to have an effect. Dose is between 10 and 100 mcg as an intravenous bolus.
- A weaker solution can be prepared by diluting 1 mL of the 1:10 000 preparation up to 10 mL with saline. You can use this weaker solution to bolus 1 mL (10 mcg) aliquots initially and increase according to response.
- During cardiac arrest the mini-jet is used.
- For infusions put 5 mg into 50 mL saline (100 mcg/mL) and commence at 5 mL/hour then adjust according to response. It is most useful for hypotension resistant to other treatments (e.g. in septic shock) and where a significant component of myocardial depression exists.
- Adrenaline can also be nebulised (5 mg per dose – 5 mL of 1:1000 repeated every 15–30 minutes) for bronchospasm and airway oedema associated with anaphylaxis and croup.

Dobutamine

Dobutamine is a direct-acting β_1 agonist giving positive inotropy and chronotropy and a resulting increase in CO. It also has β_2 and α effects that give some splanchnic vasodilatation and a reduction in SVR, peripheral vascular resistance and afterload. Consequently, BP can increase or fall. The increased CO and fall in afterload make it an ideal agent for low CO states.

- Its main uses are therefore in cardiogenic shock, sepsis with low CO, heart failure and following myocardial infarction.
- It may be used in combination with noradrenaline to increase BP – especially in sepsis.
- It increases atrioventricular node conduction and myocardial oxygen consumption and therefore its use may be limited by excessive tachycardias, arrhythmias and myocardial ischaemia.
- It is important to ensure the patient is adequately fluid loaded prior to use, especially in sepsis.
- Its use is contraindicated where there is cardiac outflow obstruction (e.g. aortic stenosis) and caution must be taken where the patient is taking MAOIs or tricyclic antidepressants or has any pre-existing arrhythmia.

Dilution

- Vials contain 250 mcg in 5 mL (50 mcg/mL).
- Put 250 mcg into 50 mL saline (5 mcg/mL) and start at 2 mL/hour (1–7 mL/hour).

Dopamine

Dopamine is a naturally occurring catecholamine, which agonises β_1, β_2, α and dopamine receptors.

- At low doses dopamine behaves like dobutamine, with an increased CO although with less tachycardia.
- SVR may initially reduce but as the dose increases, so does the α-mediated vasoconstriction, and SVR and BP tends to increase.
- Both its β_2 and dopamine receptor effects cause a degree of renal and splanchnic vasodilatation; however, there is no evidence that this leads to any renal protection. The rise in CO and reduction of sodium absorption in the kidneys leads to an increase in urine output.
- It can cause arrhythmias and myocardial ischaemia.
- The onset is within 5 minutes. Its effects last 10 minutes, with a half-life of 2 minutes, and it therefore needs to be given by infusion.

Dilution

- Vials contain 200 mg in 5 mL (40 mg/mL).
- Dilute into 50 mL (4 mg/mL) with saline and start at 2 mL/hour (range 1–9 mL/hour).

Milrinone

A phosphodiesterase inhibitor, milrinone increases cyclic adenosine monophosphate levels leading to a positive inotropic action to increase cardiac contractility and output. The increase in cyclic adenosine monophosphate also causes vasodilatation and an improvement in the ability of the heart to relax (and therefore fill) during diastole. This makes the drug ideal for use in low-output cardiac failure to improve contractility, to off-load the heart and to improve relaxation and filling.

- It reduces ventricular wall tension and increases coronary perfusion and therefore causes little or no increase in myocardial oxygen consumption or work.
- The hypotension caused may be significant and patients frequently require additional noradrenaline for BP support.
- Arrhythmias may also result and caution must be taken in patients with cardiomyopathy or outflow obstruction.

Dilution

- Vials contain 10 mg in 10 mL.
- Dilute 10 mg into 50 mL normal saline (0.2 mg/mL) and start at 5 mL/hour (range 5–10 mL/hour).

DRUGS TO TREAT BRADYCARDIA

Both atropine and glycopyrrolate are competitive antagonists at muscarinic receptors that act to block vagal parasympathetic stimulation. They produce a tachycardia by blocking vagal slowing of the heart. They also block vagal activity throughout the body and therefore reduce gut motility and secretions (including saliva), cause bronchodilatation and reduced airway secretions, inhibit sweating and cause urinary retention.

TABLE 18.3 A comparison of the effects of adrenaline, dobutamine, dopamine and milrinone

	Adrenaline	Dobutamine	Dopamine	Milrinone
Action	Potent β_1, β_2, α agonist	Mainly β_1 agonist, β_2 and α agonist also	Agonist at β_1, β_2, α, dopamine receptors	Synthetic PDE inhibitor
Predominant effects	Increased cardiac contractility and rate, increased SVR and BP (at higher doses), bronchodilatation	Increased CO and HR, reduced SVR, PVR and afterload BP may rise or fall	Increased CO and HR Effect on SVR and BP depends on dose (increase as dose increases)	Increased CO, increase diastolic relaxation, lowers BP
Other actions	Increased PVR, increased HR, increased myocardial oxygen consumption	Increased myocardial oxygen demand and AV node conduction	Increased coronary perfusion and myocardial oxygen consumption	Minimal effects on HR and myocardial work
Main uses	Low cardiac output states and severe hypotension, cardiac arrest, bronchoconstriction and anaphylaxis	Low cardiac output states associated with heart failure, sepsis and post myocardial infarct	Low CO states, especially where splanchnic blood flow is compromised	Low cardiac output heart failure
Dose and dilution	1 mL 1:1000 = 1 mg 10 mL 1:10 000 = 1 mg (100 mcg/mL) Bolus: 10–100 mcg intravenously Infusion: 5 mg in 50 mL start at 5 mL/hour Nebuliser: 5 mL of 1:1000	Vial: 250 mcg in 5 mL Put 250 mcg into 50 mL saline (5 mg/mL) Start at 2 mL/hour (1–7 mL/ hour)	Vial: 200 mg in 5 mL (40 mg/ mL) Put 200 mg into 50 mL saline (4 mg/mL) Start at 2 mL/hour (1–9 mL/ hour)	Vial: 10 mg in 10 mL Dilute: 10 mg into 50 mL saline (0.2 mg/mL) Start: 5 mL/hour (5–10 mL/ hour)

	Adrenaline	Dobutamine	Dopamine	Milrinone
Can be given . . .	Centrally Peripherally in an emergency	Centrally Peripherally in an emergency	Centrally only	Centrally only
Pharmacokinetics	Hepatic metabolism with urinary excretion Some metabolites are active Onset is rapid (1–2 minutes) and effects can last up to 30 minutes	Hepatic metabolism Half-life is 2 minutes; therefore, must be given by infusion	25% is converted to noradrenaline at nerve terminals Rest metabolised by liver, kidneys and in plasma with renal excretion	Hepatic metabolism and renal excretion – reduce dose in renal failure Effects last 30–90 minutes
Unwanted effects	Tachycardia, arrhythmias, splanchnic vasoconstriction, hypokalaemia, hyperglycaemia	Tachycardia and arrhythmias, myocardial ischaemia	Significant nausea, tachycardia, dysrhythmias and angina Renal, splanchnic vasoconstriction at high doses	Hypotension – often requires noradrenaline support Arrhythmias, nausea
Caution	Elderly, hypovolaemic, use with halothane or isoflurane Increased action with MAOIs/TCAs	Not for use with cardiac outflow obstruction Increased action with MAOIs/TCAs	Hypovolaemia, ischaemic heart disease, arrhythmias Increased action with MAOIs/TCAs	Stenotic valve disease and cardiomyopathy Ischaemic heart disease Caution with MAOIs

PDE, phosphodiesterase; SVR, systemic vascular resistance; BP, blood pressure; CO, cardiac output; HR, heart rate; PVR, peripheral vascular resistance; AV, atrioventricular; MAOI, monoamine oxidase inhibitor; TCA, tricyclic antidepressant

Atropine

Atropine causes a profound vagal block and is more useful for profound bradycardias. It can cause central anticholinergic syndrome (*see* Table 18.4).

Glycopyrrolate

Glycopyrrolate doesn't cross the blood–brain barrier, preventing central effects. It causes fewer arrhythmias than atropine, and it is superior at reducing salivary secretions. It is more versatile in graduated doses. It has a slower onset of action (within 3 minutes) than atropine and causes a less profound vagal block.

TABLE 18.4 A comparison of the effects of atropine and glycopyrrolate

	Atropine	Glycopyrrolate
Main actions	↑HR (++++), ↓saliva (++)	↑HR (+++), ↓saliva (+++++)
Vials and dilution	1 mL vials containing either 500 or 600 mcg Draw up neat 3 mg mini-jet for arrest situations	Either 600 or 200 mcg/mL in either 1 mL or 3 mL vials (check carefully) Drawn up neat
Dose	Adult dose is 500–600 mcg intravenously Paediatric dose is 20 mcg/kg intravenously 3 mg in adults causes complete vagal blockade (further doses have no effect) It is an 'all or nothing' drug and doses less than 500 mcg can cause a bradycardia	Adult dose for bradycardia is 200–600 mcg bolus (starting with 200 mcg) Paediatric dose is 4–10 mcg/kg As a pre-medication, glycopyrrolate can be given to reduce secretions
Pharmacokinetics	50% protein bound and moderately distributed Hepatic metabolism, renal excretion Half-life is 2.5 hours	Rapid redistribution from the plasma within 5 minutes, although effects can last for 2–3 hours 80% of the drug is excreted unchanged renally Some hepatic metabolism
Side effects	Dry mouth, urinary retention, inhibition of sweating	
	↓Atrioventricular conduction time and dysrhythmias	Headache and drowsiness
	Central anticholinergic syndrome: confusion, agitation, hallucinations and somnolence – especially in the elderly	

HR, heart rate

DRUGS TO REDUCE THE BLOOD PRESSURE

Occasionally you may need to reduce the BP intra-operatively. Although several drugs can be used for this specific indication, it is usually easier and faster to give a bolus of anaesthetic agent or to increase the volatile agent used. If additional agents are required it is best to use a short-acting drug and assess response.

β BLOCKERS
Esmolol
- Esmolol is a cardioselective β_1 antagonist causing bradycardia and hypotension within 5–10 minutes.
- Short acting: metabolised by red blood cell esterases, its action lasts 15–20 minutes.
- Caution in asthma, heart failure, heart block and drugs prolonging atrioventricular conduction (e.g. verapamil). It can also prolong the action of suxamethonium.

Dilution
- Usually 10 mg/mL. Give a 25 mg bolus and observe effect. Can give further boluses up to 100 mg. Infusions can be given at 15–150 mcg/kg/minute.
- Vials may also contain 250 mg/mL – check carefully.

Labetolol
- Labetolol is a longer-acting non-selective α and β antagonist. It lasts 2–4 hours.
- Give in 5 mg boluses up to 100 mg. Go slowly: labetolol takes 5–30 minutes to have an effect and so too much can be given easily.

Dilution
- Vials contain 5 mg/mL. Infusions of 20–160 mg/hour (4–30 mL/hour) can be given for a continued effect.
- Cautions as for esmolol.

Glycerine trinitrate
- Glycerine trinitrate is a nitrate compound causing primarily venodilatation with additional arterial vasodilatation, especially at higher doses.
- It reduces the BP, SVR, central venous pressure and myocardial oxygen demand and therefore can be used to treat hypertension, angina and cardiac failure.
- Sublingually metered sprays deliver 400 mcg per spray. The dose is two sprays. Action occurs within a few minutes and lasts for up to 30 minutes.
- Intravenously an infusion of 10–200 mcg/minute can be given. Intravenous solution needs to be protected from light. Onset is between 1–2 minutes.

DRUGS TO TREAT BRONCHOCONSTRICTION
Salbutamol
- Salbutamol is a β_2 agonist.
- It can be given via a nebuliser (2.5–5 mg maximally every 15 minutes) or by metered dose inhaler. Ten puffs can be delivered into the endotracheal tube; this generally has better distribution to the lower airways than the nebulised form.
- Vials of the intravenous preparation contain 50–500 mcg/mL and so care needs to be taken when drawing up.

- For severe bronchospasm a slow intravenous bolus of 250 mcg over 5–10 minutes should be given, followed by an infusion.
- Dilute 1 mg in 50 mL to make 20 mcg/mL. Run at 15–60 mL/hour and do not exceed 0.5 mcg/kg/minute.
- There may be a slight reduction of BP from β_2 effects at low doses, although its main side effects are to cause tachycardia and potentially arrhythmias via β_1 stimulation and these may well limit its use. Anxiety, tremors, palpitations and hypokalaemia are all common side effects.

Magnesium

Magnesium is commonly used as a bronchodilator, an antiarrhythmic agent and to reduce seizures in pre-eclampsia. It is a cofactor for multiple enzyme reactions and it reduces acetylcholine release from nerve terminals, although its exact mechanism of action is uncertain.

- It slows conduction in the heart and prologues the PR interval and atrioventricular node refractory periods, as well as causing bronchodilatation and vasodilatation.
- Its main side effects are hypotension, muscle weakness and drowsiness. Levels may need to be monitored in prolonged treatment.
- Vials contain a 50% solution of magnesium sulphate containing 2 mmol/mL (0.5 mg/mL).
- For both asthma and arrhythmias give 2 g (equal to 8 mmol or 4 mL). Dilute up to 20 mL and give as a slow intravenous bolus over 10–20 minutes.

Aminophylline

Aminophylline is a phosphodiesterase inhibitor, similar to milrinone, with some positive inotropic and chronotropic actions. Used in refractory bronchospasm, its increased side effect profile includes arrhythmias, reduced seizure threshold and reduced SVR and BP.

- It is given orally in the community (theophylline) and has a narrow therapeutic range (10–20 mcg/mL plasma level), above which significant arrhythmias and seizures occur.
- If the patient is not already on theophylline then load with 5 mg/kg slowly over 10–15 minutes with full electrocardiograph and BP monitoring. Following this, start an infusion at 0.5 mg/kg/hour.

DRUGS FOR TACHYARRHYTHMIAS

Several drugs may be used for tachyarrhythmias and this will depend on the underlying heart rhythm.

Magnesium

Magnesium helps to stabilise the myocardium and can be useful when given as an adjunct to treatment in patients with frequent ectopics, atrial fibrillation or flutter as well as other ventricular tachycardias. If the arrhythmia is relatively benign in an otherwise stable patient, magnesium may be the only drug required alongside searching for and treating the cause.

In supraventricular tachyarrhythmias without BP compromise a short-acting β blocker may be tried (e.g. esmolol or labetolol, as described earlier).

Adenosine

Adenosine acts directly on adenosine receptors in the heart to reduce sinoatrial and atrioventricular node conduction.

- A transient slowing of atrial activity and slowing of ventricular response occurs, which reveals the underlying atrial rhythm and potentially terminates a supraventricular tachycardia.
- Adenosine acts in 10 seconds and lasts 10–20 seconds.
- In the awake patient, transient facial flushing, dyspnoea and chest pain are common. Bronchospasm may be seen and caution must be used in asthmatics.
- The dose is a 3 mg rapid bolus followed by a 6 mg bolus, a further 6 mg bolus and then a 12 mg bolus at 1- to 2-minute intervals until a response is seen.

Amiodarone

Amiodarone is a class III antiarrhythmic agent used for both supraventricular and ventricular arrhythmias.

- Initially a loading dose of 5 mg/kg is given (generally 300 mg in an adult) given over an hour. Following this an infusion of 900 mg is given over 24 hours if the arrhythmia persists.
- For a compromising rhythm the initial 300 mg of amiodarone may be given over 20 minutes, although monitor closely for severe hypotension and bradycardia.
- It can cause hypotension, bradycardias and significant arrhythmias especially if the patient is hypokalaemic. It is extremely irritant to veins and therefore given centrally if possible or via a large-bore peripheral cannula.

DRUGS USED SPECIFICALLY FOR ANAESTHESIA

The following drugs are used specifically in anaesthesia; however, their use is rare. They are generally stored in a central location in the theatre complex, often in the recovery room.

Intralipid (intravenous lipid emulsion)

Intralipid is given in cases of local anaesthetic toxicity to reduce the harmful cardio-vascular effects.

- It comes as a pre-prepared 20% solution and is given as an initial bolus dose, which is repeated at 5-minute intervals, as well as a simultaneous infusion.
- The initial bolus dose is 1.5 mg/kg over 1 minute with a simultaneous infusion started at 15 mL/kg/hour (1000 mL/hour for a 70 kg patient).
- The bolus doses can be repeated at 5-minute intervals to a maximum of three boluses.
- The infusion rate can also be doubled to 30 mL/kg/hour (2000 mL/hour for a 70 kg patient) after 5 minutes if there is no cardiovascular improvement. The infusion is continued until there is improvement or a total dose of 12 mL/kg has been given (e.g. 840 mL total dose for a 70 kg patient).

Dantrolene

Dantrolene is a drug used for malignant hyperthermia. It acts on the sarcoplasmic reticulum (inhibiting the ryanodine receptor) in skeletal muscle to reduce calcium ion release and thus decrease the damaging global muscle contractions.

- Vials contain dantrolene 20 mg plus mannitol 3 g and sodium hydroxide: it needs to be made up with 60 mL of sterile water.
- For malignant hyperthermia an initial dose of 1 mg/kg intravenously (approximately four vials) is given followed by repeated doses up to 10 mg/kg (average requirement is 2–3 mg/kg).
- This is difficult to dissolve and will require a large volume of sterile water and so is best made up in a large sterile theatre dish. It has a pH of 9.5 and causes tissue necrosis with extravasation.

Key points

- You will frequently have to use emergency drugs as part of your anaesthetic practice and emergency resuscitation.
- Learn the autonomic nervous system in detail before learning all of the drugs individually – this will give you an integrated approach.
- You must know these drugs in detail and you must know how to prepare them and how to infuse them.
- While life-saving, many have serious side effects that you must be able to recognise and prevent.

CHAPTER 19

NCEPOD categories and anaesthetic implications

NICK DOREE

WHAT IS NCEPOD?

NCEPOD stands for the National Confidential Enquiry into Patient Outcome and Death. It has been renamed from the National Confidential Enquiry into Perioperative Deaths, which was established in 1988.

As the name suggests, the initial focus of this organisation was on anaesthetic and surgical practice but it now encompasses all specialties.

The purpose of the organisation is ultimately to improve standards of patient care. It collates information on various aspects of clinical practice, expertly reviews the evidence and identifies potentially remediable aspects of care that are considered substandard. Reports, which are widely available to clinicians, are then generated, making various recommendations for improvements in healthcare.

NCEPOD CLASSIFICATION OF INTERVENTIONS

In 2004 NCEPOD defined the urgency of surgery or interventions into four main categories. The purpose of this is to:

- inform clinicians and managers of lists and allow prioritisation
- check that patients are operated on within an appropriate time frame for their condition
- check that only appropriate operations are undertaken out of hours.[1]

The category of urgency of surgery should be defined when a case is booked for theatre. It should be agreed between the surgeon booking the case and the anaesthetist being informed of the case. There can occasionally be grey areas that may lead to contention.

The four main categories

1. *Immediate*: immediate life-, limb- or organ-saving intervention.
2. *Urgent*: intervention for potentially life- or limb-threatening conditions.

3. *Expedited*: patient requiring early intervention where the condition is not a threat to life, limb or organ.
4. *Elective*: intervention booked in advance of admission to hospital.

ANAESTHETIC IMPLICATIONS

The urgency of surgery has implications for timing of surgery, preoperative assessment and investigations, conduct of anaesthesia and post-operative care.

Immediate

- For example, ruptured abdominal aortic aneurysm, acute extradural haematoma, major abdominal or thoracic trauma, fracture with neurovascular deficit
- Next available theatre slot
- Intervention should proceed within 1 hour
- Resuscitation takes place simultaneously with intervention or surgery
- Proceed even if patient not fasted

Depending on the condition, the patient may be inherently unstable and the focus is on the intervention or surgery that will stabilise the patient. There is limited time available for preoperative assessment and investigations.

- An ABCDE (Airway, Breathing, Circulation, Disability, Exposure) approach is likely to be used or a primary survey as taught by advanced trauma life support.
- Large-bore intravenous access is secured, with bloods sent for full blood count, urea and electrolytes, clotting, cross-match and fluid resuscitation initiated.
- History may be limited but basic information on past medical history, previous anaesthetics and problems, drugs, allergies and airway assessment can usually be quickly elucidated.

Patients may require their airway securing before transfer to theatre and theatre may need preparing for major blood loss with invasive lines run through with warming devices and rapid infusing devices prepared.

Induction of anaesthesia will destabilise the patient further and may need to be undertaken in theatre with the surgeon scrubbed and ready. More cardiovascularly stable induction agents should be used and doses reduced. A rapid sequence induction will be required with an experienced, senior anaesthetist. A second or third pair of hands can be invaluable. Invasive monitoring will be required but may need to be inserted after surgery has begun.

The majority of these cases will require critical care post-operatively.

Urgent

- For example, perforated bowel with peritonitis, compound fracture, critical limb ischaemia
- Emergency list (including at night)
- Intervention should usually proceed within hours of decision to operate
- Full resuscitation should be complete prior to intervention
- Patient should be fasted

Within this category some cases will be more urgent than others and some hospitals subdivide this further (e.g. within 6 hours and within 24 hours).

Although surgery is urgent, full resuscitation of the patient should have taken place prior to induction of anaesthesia to prevent unnecessary instability.

There is time for full history, examination and case note review with basic investigations such as electrocardiograph, blood tests, blood gases, X-rays and echocardiography.

Anaesthesia can be planned with appropriate monitoring and seniority of anaesthetist. Any invasive monitoring can be placed pre-induction.

Critical care will frequently be required post-operatively.

Expedited

- Wide range of surgical procedures in stable or non-septic patients (e.g. tendon or nerve injuries, bowel tumour starting to obstruct, retinal detachment)
- Emergency or elective list with spare capacity (not at night)
- Intervention usually within days of decision to operate
- Any resuscitation required complete

As with urgent cases there is time for relevant investigations required, such as echocardiography or pulmonary function testing. There is also time for other speciality input if required.

These are not emergency cases and should not be undertaken at night (the cut-off time is usually considered to be 22.00 hours), when hospital staffing is at reduced levels. Theatre should be reserved and ready for emergency and urgent cases.

Elective

- All conditions not classified as emergency, urgent or expedited (e.g. elective abdominal aortic aneurysm repair, joint replacements, laparoscopic cholecystectomy, tonsillectomy)
- Elective lists
- Intervention pre-planned and done at a time to suit hospital and patient

Obviously, elective cases should be fully worked up for theatre. Medical conditions optimised, operations postponed because of significant intercurrent illness and specialist input received if required.

There is time for more specialised investigations such as cardiopulmonary exercise testing or coronary angiography. Occasionally there may even be an indication for an operation such as aortic valve replacement prior to the original planned operation. The anaesthetist should assess high-risk cases weeks in advance so risk stratification can be done and discussed with the patient.

Post-operative critical care beds should be pre-booked and explained to the patient.

Key points
- Emergency and elective cases are very different situations.
- The emergency case requires a certain degree of 'belt and braces' approach, while the elective case requires meticulous assessment and preparation.
- The grading of severity allows the optimisation of patient care and the allocation of resources.

REFERENCE

1. National Confidential Enquiry into Patient Outcome and Death (NCEPOD). *Revised Classification of Intervention 2004* www.ncepod.org.uk/pdf/NCEPODClassification.pdf. Accessed 18/04/2013.

CHAPTER 20

The pregnant patient

SOPHIE BISHOP

It is unlikely that when you start anaesthetics that you will spend much time on the labour ward. However, you may still come across a pregnant patient requiring non-obstetric surgery or in the emergency department, and there are some important considerations to be aware of when looking after these women.

In order to provide safe anaesthesia for the mother and foetus, it is essential to know about the physiological changes that characterise the three trimesters of pregnancy.

PHYSIOLOGICAL CHANGES OF PREGNANCY

Most physiological changes occur in response to the increased metabolic demands of the uterus, placenta and foetus. The main physiological changes that influence anaesthesia and resuscitation of the pregnant woman are discussed here.

Cardiovascular

- Aortocaval compression is the compression of the great vessels against the vertebral bodies by the gravid uterus in the supine position from 20 weeks' gestation onwards.
- Venacaval compression reduces venous return and cardiac output with a compensatory increase in systemic vascular resistance. This might be symptomless or associated with hypotension.
- Reduced placental blood flow may result from the reduced cardiac output, vasoconstriction and compression of the aorta.
- Tilting the mother by 30 degrees, usually to the left, improves placental flow.
- Physiological anaemia of pregnancy – the plasma volume increases by 45% but the red cell mass increases by 20%. This results in a fall in haemoglobin concentration to about 12 g/dL at term.
- Increased cardiac output and decreased systemic vascular resistance is a result of both an increase in heart rate and stroke volume.
- Ejection systolic murmurs are common.

Respiratory

- Capillary engorgement and oedema of the upper airway (so avoid nasal tubes), in combination with enlarged breasts and increased thoracic circumference can make intubation more difficult with a standard Macintosh blade.

- The incidence of failed intubation is much higher in the pregnant population, peaking in the third trimester.
- There is a reduction in the functional residual capacity by 20%. This results in reduced oxygen reserves, so pre-oxygenation is less effective and desaturation is likely to occur much faster than in the non-pregnant patient.
- There is an increase in both respiratory rate and tidal volume, which is due to an increased sensitivity to CO_2 mediated by progesterone. This results in a fall in $PaCO_2$, to about 4.1 kPa.

Gastrointestinal

- Gastro-oesophageal reflux occurs in a least 80% of women caused by the effects of progesterone reducing the lower oesophageal sphincter tone and the uterus pushing the stomach into a horizontal position. The time of onset is considered to be from 16–20 weeks onwards.
- Gastric emptying is probably normal apart from during labour.

Coagulation

- Pregnancy induces a hypercoagulable state, with many changes in the clotting system, which are not reflected in routine tests.

SURGERY FOR THE PREGNANT PATIENT

It is estimated that 1%–2% of pregnant women require incidental surgery during their pregnancy (appendicitis, ovarian torsion and trauma are common indications). Surgery is associated with a greater risk of abortion, growth restriction and low birth weight, although these problems probably result from the primary disease rather than the anaesthetic or surgery itself. Elective surgery should not be performed at all during pregnancy. Non-urgent surgery is usually delayed until the second trimester because of the possible risk of teratogenic effects on the foetus (greatest during the period of organogenesis, which continues to the twelfth gestational week). Emergency surgery will proceed regardless of gestational age to preserve the life of the mother.

The goals of providing anaesthesia to these patients:
- optimise and maintain normal maternal physiological function
- optimise and maintain utero-placental blood flow and oxygen delivery
- avoid unwanted drug effects on the foetus
- avoid stimulating the myometrium
- avoid awareness during general anaesthesia
- use regional anaesthesia if possible.

General considerations

There should be a multidisciplinary approach with senior involvement including the obstetricians. Foetal well-being should be assessed by ultrasound or Doppler before and after anaesthesia and surgery. Once foetal viability is assumed (24–26 weeks) the foetal heart rate should be monitored; this may be difficult in obese patients or during abdominal surgery.

Preoperatively

- Electrocardiograph changes during pregnancy are caused by the cephalad displacement of the diaphragm by the uterus and result in left axis deviation and non-specific ST and T wave changes.
- Foetal exposure during radiological investigations should be minimised.
- Blood results should be available, and blood cross-matched for major surgery.
- Premedication should include aspiration prophylaxis from the second trimester onwards (e.g. ranitidine, sodium citrate and metoclopramide).
- Remember deep venous thrombosis prophylaxis, as pregnant patients are hypercoagulable.

Intra-operatively

- Airway management should involve a rapid sequence induction from approximately 16 weeks onwards. However, if the patient is symptomatic or has additional risk factors for regurgitation, perform a rapid sequence induction earlier.
- The advantages of regional anaesthesia are that it involves minimal foetal drug exposure and the mother maintains her own airway.
- If using a general anaesthetic, even though anaesthetic requirements are reduced in pregnancy, it is important to use adequate doses to prevent awareness and the associated catecholamine release that will reduce placental blood flow.
- From 20 weeks' gestation, remember to use a 30-degree left lateral tilt to reduce aortocaval compression, as in the supine position. This compromises uterine blood flow, even though blood pressure might give a normal reading on the upper limb. The effect of regional or general anaesthesia is to abolish the normal compensatory mechanisms and the situation is exacerbated. Using an operating table that tilts is the best option; other options are to insert a wedge under the right side or, lastly, manual displacement of the uterus.
- Treat haemorrhage aggressively; avoid hypovolaemia and anaemia, as both affect foetal oxygenation.

Post-operatively

- Good and effective post-operative analgesia is essential to reduce maternal catecholamine secretion. For minor surgery paracetamol and codeine with local anaesthesia may be used.
- Avoid non-steroidal anti-inflammatory drugs.
- For major surgery regional anaesthesia may be preferential.
- The other concern in the post-operative phase is the risk of premature labour, so women should be told to report any uterine contractions in order that tocolytic treatment can be started if necessary.

RESUSCITATION OF THE PREGNANT PATIENT

If you ever have to put out a cardiac arrest call for a pregnant patient, it is important to state that it is a 'maternal cardiac arrest'. Most hospitals have a designated maternal cardiac arrest team, which will include the obstetricians and the neonatologists.

Fortunately, maternal cardiac arrest is rare; resuscitation follows the adult algorithms as described in the advanced trauma and life support protocols. The important differences between adult cardiac arrest and maternal cardiac arrest are highlighted here.

Left lateral tilt

After 20 weeks' gestation the mother must be tilted at the start of resuscitation to relieve aortocaval compression. This can be done using a wedge, a pillow or your knees, depending where you are.

Early intubation

Early intubation is important, to aid oxygen delivery because of both decreased oxygen reserves and higher oxygen demands and to prevent aspiration of gastric contents. We have already discussed the increased chance of a difficult intubation, so call for senior anaesthetic help early.

Perimortem caesarean section

After 20 weeks' gestation, the foetus should be delivered. It improves the likelihood of successful resuscitation of the mother. It should be commenced within 4 minutes of cardiac arrest and completed within 5 minutes of cardiac arrest. There will be none or minimal bleeding, so there is no need to transfer the woman to theatre; a scalpel is the only equipment required. A perimortem caesarean section may also save the baby.

Cause of cardiac arrest

During resuscitation it is important to consider the reversible causes of cardiac arrest. In the pregnant population the following are common causes of maternal cardiac arrest.
- Thromboembolism:
  > pulmonary embolism
  > amniotic fluid embolism.
- Toxins:
  > local anaesthetic toxicity
  > hypermagnesaemia.
- Hypovolaemia:
  > haemorrhage
  > sepsis.
- Other known risk factors:
  > pre-existing cardiac disease (myocardial infarction)
  > hypertensive disease of pregnancy (intracranial haemorrhage).

Key points
- Difficult intubation is more common in pregnancy.
- Oxygen desaturation is more rapid in pregnant women.
- There is a high risk of gastric aspiration.
- The clinical signs of hypovolaemia may be masked by the physiological changes of pregnancy.
- Regional anaesthesia should be used in preference to general anaesthesia where appropriate.
- If possible, surgery should be delayed until the second trimester.
- Ensure a 30-degree tilt, then use the ABC approach during cardiac arrest.
- Perform a perimortem caesarean section during cardiac arrest after 20 weeks' gestation.

FURTHER READING

- Heidemann B, McClure J. Changes in maternal physiology during pregnancy. *Cont Educ Anaesth Crit Pain.* 2003; **3**(3): 65–8.
- Walton N, Melachuri V. Anaesthesia for non-obstetric surgery during pregnancy. *Cont Educ Anaesth Crit Pain.* 2006; **6**(2): 83–5.

CHAPTER 21

The obese patient

GILLIAN CAMPBELL

Obesity is increasing in prevalence – 20% of adults in the UK are obese and 1% are morbidly obese. Obesity is classified according to body mass index (BMI).

$$BMI = weight\ (kg)/height^2\ (m^2)$$

World Health Organization classification:
- Normal: BMI 18–24.9 kg/m²
- Overweight: BMI 25–29.9 kg/m²
- Obese: BMI 30–39.9 kg/m²
- Morbidly obese: BMI >40 kg/m² or BMI >35 kg/m² with associated co-morbidities
- Super morbidly obese: BMI >55 kg/m²

Obesity affects every body system and is a contributory factor to many other diseases. It can cause particular difficulties for the anaesthetist.

HOW DOES OBESITY AFFECT THE AIRWAY?

Bag and mask ventilation
- It can be difficult to maintain a good seal with a face mask, and higher airway pressures (due to increased weight on the chest wall) are often required for effective ventilation.
- Airway obstruction is common – have a low threshold for airway adjuncts. Ask about obstructive sleep apnoea.

Laryngeal mask ventilation
- Insertion of the laryngeal mask is not usually problematic; however, it is often difficult to maintain satisfactory ventilation while breathing spontaneously.
- As higher airway pressures are often required during positive pressure ventilation it is sometimes difficult to have adequate seal around the laryngeal mask for effective ventilation.
- It is generally better to intubate obese patients for even the shortest procedures.
- As a rule of thumb, if when lying flat the patient's belly is above his or her nose, intubate.

Intubation

- It is essential that a full airway assessment is performed preoperatively (*see* Chapter 9).
- Difficulties include:
  - › large breasts making insertion of laryngoscope awkward
  - › a tendency to oesophageal reflux, necessitating a rapid sequence induction
  - › early and rapid oxygen desaturation.
- It can be difficult to obtain correct 'sniffing morning air' position and many clinicians now advocate the 'ramped position'.

HOW DOES OBESITY AFFECT THE RESPIRATORY SYSTEM?

- The most important physiological effect is the reduction of the functional residual capacity (FRC) because of abdominal fat pushing upwards on the diaphragm.
- At the end of expiration and acts as an oxygen reservoir after pre-oxygenation.
- Decreased FRC means that there is a reduction in this reserve for the body to utilise during decreased ventilation or physiological stress.
- This makes pre-oxygenation particularly important, although less effective.
- Obese patients have an increased basal metabolic rate, which when combined with a lower FRC means that their oxygen saturations drop very quickly.

HOW DOES OBESITY AFFECT THE CARDIOVASCULAR SYSTEM?

- Occult cardiovascular disease is common with hypertension and ischaemic heart disease particularly prevalent.
- Intravenous access can be very difficult.
- Cardiovascular monitors are less accurate and reliable, particularly non-invasive blood pressure. An arterial line maybe required.
- They will have a larger circulating volume.

HOW DO OBESE PATIENTS HANDLE DRUGS?

- Drug handling is affected by changes in volume of distribution, plasma protein binding and clearance.
- Fat-soluble drugs such should be calculated on ideal body weight.
- Less fat soluble on ideal weight plus 20%.
- Suxamethonium should be calculated on total body weight.
- Particular care should be taken with opiates. Obstructive sleep apnoea (OSA) is common in obese patients and relatively underdiagnosed. Careful preoperative enquiry is important, as patients with OSA are often very sensitive to opiates and they should be administered with caution.

HOW DOES OBESITY AFFECT OTHER SYSTEMS?

- Gastrointestinal: gastro-oesophageal reflux is more common, liver disease can occur.
- Haematological: higher risk of venous thromboembolism.
- Endocrine: type 2 diabetes mellitus is more common.
- Musculoskeletal: osteoarthritis is common.

THE 'IDEAL ANAESTHETIC'

Senior help is required for morbidly obese patients. You will also require more staff for positioning. You should have enough staff available so that you could urgently roll the patient into the lateral position. In very obese patients this may be five people.

Preoperative assessment

Routine preoperative assessment with particular attention to:

- airway assessment – Mallampati, neck extension, collar size, snoring
- symptoms of OSA – daytime somnolence, falling asleep at inappropriate times, morning headaches
- gastrointestinal reflux
- concomitant disease – ischaemic heart disease, hypertension and diabetes
- exercise tolerance
- ensure adequate thromboprophylaxis.

Induction

- Position your patient appropriately – if the patient is very heavy it may be best to anaesthetise him or her on the operating table to avoid any transfers. Remember to check that the patient does not exceed the maximum weight for the table.
- Ensure that monitor readings are reliable. Use an appropriately sized blood pressure cuff. If you are unable to obtain satisfactory readings, invasive monitoring may be required. Ensure electrocardiograph electrodes are placed correctly, as low complexes are often seen because of depth of subcutaneous tissue.
- Pre-oxygenate for 3 minutes with a well-fitting mask until the expired oxygen concentration is >80%.
- Induction drugs will be your personal preference but they may need a rapid sequence induction.
- Have the difficult intubation trolley handy.
- Confirm tube position visually (both sides of the chest rising and falling), by capnography and auscultation.

Intra-operatively

- Positioning – take special care protecting pressure areas.
- Give adequate analgesia but avoid large doses of opiates.
- Be aware that surgery may be technically difficult and may take longer.

Emergence

- This can be the riskiest time for the patient.
- It is vital that the muscle relaxation is fully reversed. Always use a nerve stimulator.
- Sit the patient upright.
- Wait until the patient is fully awake, fully reversed, obeying commands and breathing adequately before extubating.
- It is safer to extubate on a trolley rather than the bed, as the patient will be easier to manoeuvre should any complications occur.

Recovery

- Administer supplemental oxygen, which may be required for an extended period.
- Titrate analgesia as required.
- Obese patients are more likely to require level 2 care post-operatively.

Key points

- Senior assistance is required for morbidly obese patients.
- Obese airways are often difficult to manage.
- Have a low threshold for intubating patients.
- The reduction in FRC means that oxygen desaturation occurs quickly.
- Pre-oxygenation is essential.
- Concomitant diseases are common.
- Take care with opiates.
- Extubate fully awake, fully reversed and breathing adequately.

FURTHER READING

- Lotia S, Bellamy MC. Anaesthesia and morbid obesity. *Cont Educ Anaesth Crit Pain.* 2008; **8**(5): 151–6.

CHAPTER 22

The cardiac patient presenting for non-cardiac surgery

BALSAM ALTEMIMI

Patients with cardiac disease presenting for non-cardiac surgery are a challenge to the most senior anaesthetist. As a new starter in anaesthesia, you are not expected to manage these patients without senior advice and direct supervision.

In this chapter we will cover the following points.

- The risk assessment of patients presenting for non-cardiac surgery
- The approach to cardiac conditions that place patients at higher risk for myocardial infarction and cardiac death:
  › coronary artery disease
  › aortic stenosis.

BACKGROUND

The incidence of post-operative myocardial infarction in patients undergoing non-cardiac surgery is difficult to quantify. In patients with increased cardiac risk undergoing non-cardiac surgery the incidence of myocardial infarction is 5.1% at 30 days.[1] The incidence is much higher in patients known to have coronary artery disease scheduled for vascular surgery.[2]

It's essential that all patients are risk assessed appropriately. This will allow appropriate counselling and consent, as well as the institution of appropriate risk reduction strategies and planning for post-operative care.

Patients having elective surgery will usually have attended a preoperative assessment clinic designed to identify those at high risk.

The group presenting for urgent or emergent surgery will not have been assessed beforehand. Most of these patients will present out of hours, when the first person to see them will be the most junior member of the anaesthetic team. If faced with such a challenge, it is important to arm yourself with as much knowledge on what to look for during the preoperative assessment.

WHY ARE PATIENTS WITH CORONARY ARTERY DISEASE AT RISK OF PERIOPERATIVE ISCHAEMIA?

Both anaesthetic and surgical factors interplay to cause an imbalance between the myocardial oxygen supply and demand in at risk individuals.

- Most general anaesthetics reduce the systemic vascular resistance (SVR) and decrease myocardial contractility.
- They can also cause myocardial irritability increasing the susceptibility to arrhythmias.
- Tracheal intubation induces tachycardia and hypertension.
- Regional anaesthesia reduces the SVR through sympathetic blockade.

The stress response to surgery can lead to:

- an increase in circulating catecholamines and inflammatory mediators
- plaque instability and disruption
- hypercoagulability
- these factors can lead to coronary thrombosis and myocardial infarction.[3]

RISK ASSESSMENT

Three factors interplay in the assessment of these patients:

1. surgery-specific factors
2. patient-specific factors
3. exercise capacity or functional status.

RISK FACTORS RELATED TO SURGERY

The type of surgery plays an important part in determining risk.[4]

Note that high-risk procedures are all vascular. This is because vascular patients have the same risk factors for coronary artery disease:

- diabetes
- hypertension
- smoking
- obesity
- hyperlipidaemia
- age.

TABLE 22.1 Surgical risk of myocardial infarction and cardiac death within 30 days of surgery (modified from Boersma *et al.*[5])

Low risk, <1%	Intermediate risk, 1%–5%	High risk, >5%
Breast	Abdominal	Aortic and major vascular surgery
Dental	Carotid	Peripheral vascular surgery
Endocrine	Peripheral arterial angioplasty	
Eye	Endovascular aneurysm repair	
Gynaecology	Head and neck surgery	
Reconstructive	Neurological	
Orthopaedic – minor (knee surgery)	Orthopaedic – major (hip and spine)	
Urological – minor	Pulmonary, renal, liver transplant	
	Urological – major	

Coronary artery disease may be subclinical because activity is limited in patients with peripheral vascular disease.

Patients presenting for emergency surgery pose a high risk for cardiac complications. They will not be able to undergo any preoperative preparation and treatment of co-existing diseases.

The surgical problem can also aggravate the situation by causing:
- fluid shifts
- blood loss
- sepsis
- change in body temperature.

RISK FACTORS RELATED TO THE PATIENT
The history

This needs to be focused on uncovering risk factors known to predict the risk of non-fatal myocardial infarction and death following non-cardiac surgery. The Revised Cardiac Risk Index[6] is used to quantify risk (*see* Table 22.2).

TABLE 22.2 Revised Cardiac Risk Index[6]

Clinical risk factor	Examples
History of ischemic heart disease	Previous MI, previous positive stress test, angina, use of GTN, previous PCI or CABG, ECG Q waves
History of compensated previous congestive heart failure	Previous pulmonary oedema, third heart sound or bilateral rales, paroxysmal nocturnal dyspnoea, evidence of heart failure on chest radiograph
History of cerebrovascular disease	Previous TIA, previous stroke
Diabetes mellitus	With or without preoperative insulin therapy
Renal insufficiency	Creatinine level >177 mmol/L
High-risk surgery	Intraperitoneal, intrathoracic, or suprainguinal vascular surgery

MI, myocardial infarction; GTN, glyceryl trinitrate; PCI, percutaneous coronary intervention; CABG, coronary artery bypass graft; ECG electrocardiogram; TIA, transient ischemic attack.

Each risk factor is assigned 1 point (*see* Table 22.3).

TABLE 22.3 Classification of Revised Cardiac Risk Index – major cardiac event includes myocardial infarction, pulmonary oedema, complete heart block and cardiac arrest

Number of points	Class	Risk of major cardiac event (%)
0	I	0.4
1	II	0.9
2	III	6.6
≥3	IV	11

In addition to calculating a Revised Cardiac Risk Index score for the patient, other points in the history not to be missed include:

- identification of 'active cardiac conditions' that require evaluation and treatment before non-cardiac surgery (*see* Table 22.4)[7]
- patients with permanent pacemaker plus or minus implantable cardioverter defibrillator
- pulmonary hypertension or risk factors (e.g. chronic obstructive pulmonary disease)
- recent cardiac intervention (e.g. percutaneous coronary intervention, coronary artery bypass graft surgery)
- drug history, including antiplatelet drugs and anticoagulants with precise timing of when these drugs were stopped
- assessment of functional status begins with the history.

TABLE 22.4 Active cardiac conditions[7]

Condition	Examples
Unstable coronary syndromes	Acute or recent MI (<30 days)
	Unstable or severe angina (CCS class III or IV)
Decompensated heart failure	NYHA functional class IV
	Worsening or new-onset heart failure
Significant arrhythmias	High-grade AV block
	Symptomatic bradycardia
	Symptomatic ventricular arrhythmias
	Supraventricular arrhythmias
	AF with ventricular rate >100 bpm at rest
Severe valvular disease	Severe aortic stenosis
	Symptomatic mitral stenosis

MI, myocardial infarction; CCS, Canadian Cardiovascular Society; NYHA, New York Heart Association; AV, atrioventricular; AF, atrial fibrillation

Examination

- General appearance including, dyspnoea, cyanosis, shortness of breath at rest or during a conversation
- Heart rate and blood pressure
- Signs of heart failure (e.g. S3 gallop, raised jugular venous pressure, peripheral oedema)
- Murmurs
- Carotid bruits, peripheral pulses

Investigations

Resting electrocardiogram

An electrocardiogram (ECG) allows any changes encountered in the perioperative period to be compared with the ECG in the notes to determine if the changes are new.

In stable patients, an ECG performed within the last 30 days is acceptable.

Echocardiography

Estimating the ejection fraction with resting echocardiography is not predictive of increased risk for perioperative ischaemia, as patients with a normal ejection fraction can have significant coronary artery disease.

An echo should be reserved for:

- patients with dyspnoea of unknown origin or in patients with known symptomatic heart failure – an echo in the last 12 months is considered adequate
- patients suspected of having significant valvular heart disease.

Cardiac stress testing

Treadmill testing, radionuclide myocardial perfusion imaging and dobutamine stress echocardiography can be used to detect inducible ischaemia. Of these, dobutamine stress echocardiography is the most useful, as it has a high negative predictive value.

The indications include:

- patients with active cardiac conditions (*see* Table 22.3)
- patients with three or more of the clinical risk factors listed in Table 22.2.[6]

Cardiopulmonary exercise testing

See Chapter 4.

Coronary angiography

Coronary angiography should not be performed routinely as a risk predictor in the perioperative period. It is reserved for patients with severe symptoms or positive stress tests. Preoperative coronary artery bypass graft is indicated only in patients who require revascularisation independent of any non-cardiac surgery (*see* Table 22.4).[7]

PRACTICE GUIDELINES: PUTTING IT ALL TOGETHER

TABLE 22.5 Recommendations for preoperative revascularisation[7]

Acute coronary syndrome	High-risk NSTEMI and all STEMI
Stable angina pectoris or silent ischaemia	Left main stem CAD >50%
	Proximal LAD stenosis >50%
	2 or 3 vessel CAD with impaired LV function
	LV ischaemic area >10%
	Single remaining patent vessel with >50% stenosis and impaired LV function
Persistent ischaemia or high cardiac risk for high-risk vascular surgery	

STEMI, ST segment elevation myocardial infarction; NSTEMI, non–ST segment myocardial infarction; CAD, coronary artery disease; LAD, left anterior descending coronary artery; LV, left ventricular

PHARMACOLOGICAL THERAPIES

Optimal medical therapy is essential in high-risk patients.

β Blockers

Theoretically, β blockade should be ideal in patients at risk for perioperative ischaemia. They reduce myocardial oxygen consumption and have plaque-stabilising and anti-inflammatory properties.

The main problem is that they attenuate the physiological tachycardia in response to many perioperative events other than ischaemia (e.g. hypovolaemia, anaemia, sepsis). As a result, the only class 1 recommendation for the use of β blockers by the American College of Cardiology and the American Heart Association is:

- continuation of β blockade in patients already on β blockers
- β blockers should be started days to weeks before surgery and titrated to a target heart rate between 60 and 80 bpm.[7]

Statins

Statins have benefits beyond their lipid-lowering property; they are anti-inflammatory and stabilise coronary plaques, preventing rupture. Moreover, there is an increased mortality when statins are acutely withdrawn.[8] The recommendations are as follows:

- statins should be continued perioperatively
- statins should be started in high-risk surgery patients (between 30 days and 1 week).

Inhibitors of the renin-angiotensin system

Angiotensin-converting enzyme (ACE) inhibitors and angiotensin receptor blockers both have anti-inflammatory properties and improve endothelial function. They may help prevent ischaemia and left ventricular (LV) dysfunction.

They may cause severe hypotension under anaesthesia, which is unresponsive to vasopressors. This is avoided by stopping them for 24 hours before surgery.

The recommendations are:

- ACE inhibitors should be continued during non-cardiac surgery
- they should be started in high-risk surgery patients with LV dysfunction and considered for those having intermediate to low-risk surgery
- ACE inhibitors should be discontinued for 24 hours preoperatively in patients taking them for hypertension to avoid intra-operative hypotension, but continued when they are being taken for LV dysfunction.

Diuretics

The recommendations:

- electrolyte disturbances should be corrected
- discontinue on day of surgery in patients taking them for hypertension; continue in patients taking them for heart failure.

Antiplatelet drugs

Stopping aspirin increases the risk of ischemia. The recommendations are:

- aspirin should only be discontinued when the risk of bleeding and its consequences are high (e.g. intracranial, posterior eye chamber, prostate surgery).

For dual antiplatelet therapy, *see* 'The post–percutaneous coronary intervention patient' section later in this chapter.

ANAESTHETISING THE CARDIAC PATIENT

There are a few basic principles that should be adhered to when anaesthetising cardiac patients, and these are outlined here. Each patient must have a plan agreed and discussed by the entire team (anaesthetist, surgeon, intensivist, cardiologist).

Premedication

Benzodiazepine premedication is useful in allaying anxiety and reducing preoperative tachycardia and hypertension and should be considered for non-cardiac surgical patients unless you are concerned about respiratory function.

Monitoring

All patients should have routine monitoring as per Association of Anaesthetists of Great Britain and Ireland guidelines. In addition to this, also:
- ST segment monitoring
- invasive arterial blood pressure monitoring
- central venous catheters may be required for the administration of inotropes or vasopressors, and monitoring preload
- oesophageal Doppler cardiac output monitoring (CardioQ-ODM) has been recently recommended by the National Institute for Health and Clinical Excellence for cardiovascular monitoring in patients undergoing high-risk surgery or in any case where invasive monitoring is considered.[9]

Anaesthetic drugs

No particular drug or method has been found to be superior and the consultant will make the decision on the day. A few principles to consider are outlined here.
- Haemodynamic changes in response to induction and intubation need to be minimised.
- The use of large doses of opioids at induction is useful; however, it will delay post-operative recovery and increase length of stay on the intensive care unit.
- Etomidate is the most cardio-stable intravenous induction agent. It could be considered especially for unstable patients (e.g. a ruptured abdominal aortic aneurysm).
- Vecuronium causes the least haemodynamic disturbances compared with other non-depolarising muscle relaxants.
- Volatile anaesthetic agents have myocardial depressant effects and reduce afterload. They also have beneficial effects on the myocardium through preconditioning, where certain intracellular signal transduction pathways are activated, thus protecting the myocardium against ischaemia.
- Epidurals should be considered depending on the surgery, especially if pulmonary function is abnormal. Studies have showed no reduction in cardiac events but some reduction in pulmonary events post-operatively.[10]
- Maintenance of body temperature is essential and is associated with a lower incidence of perioperative ischaemia and arrhythmias.
- Ongoing haemodynamic monitoring and rapid correction of any volume loss is essential.

POST-OPERATIVE CARE

The need for high dependency or intensive care admission depends on a combination of patient and surgical factors, as well as functional status. In many centres using cardiopulmonary exercise testing, the results are used to decide the level of care the patient will require in the post-operative period.

For urgent or emergent cases, patients are more likely to be compromised by the presenting surgical condition as well as their co-morbidities and therefore will require a higher level of care.

Diagnosis of post-operative ischaemia is vital; the current guidelines recommend the use of trooping only in patients with ECG changes and cardiac chest pain.[6]

THE POST–PERCUTANEOUS CORONARY INTERVENTION PATIENT

Patients who have had a coronary artery bypass graft in the last 5 years and have been stable are safe to proceed with non-cardiac surgery. They usually have a lower incidence of complications. Post–percutaneous coronary intervention patients are at higher risk for cardiac events and so require special consideration.

There are two types of stents, bare metal and drug-eluting stent. They require dual anti-platelet therapy with aspirin and clopidogrel. With a bare metal stent this is 6 weeks; drug-eluting stents require 12 months because the drugs they elute slow down endothelial regrowth.

Current guidelines are as follows:

- balloon angioplasty – postpone surgery for 2 weeks
- bare metal stents – postpone surgery for 3 months (minimum 6 weeks)
- drug-eluting stents – postpone surgery for 12 months.[7]

If clopidogrel is stopped (to avoid surgical bleeding) before the minimum recommended times outlined here, the results could be catastrophic, leading to acute myocardial infarction or death. The risk of cardiac events must be balanced against the risk of surgical bleeding when managing these patients.

If the risk of bleeding is low to moderate, dual antiplatelet therapy should continue.

VALVULAR HEART DISEASE

All patients with severe valvular heart disease require clinical and echocardiographic evaluation, and, if necessary, treatment before non-cardiac surgery.[7]

Aortic stenosis

Severe aortic stenosis (AS) (defined as a valve area $<1.0\,cm^2$ with a mean transvalvular pressure gradient of $>50\,mmHg$ with a normal cardiac output) is associated with the highest risk for perioperative cardiac complications, including heart failure, non-fatal ischaemia and death.

Anaesthetising a patient with AS should be under strict haemodynamic monitoring (arterial line awake).

- The SVR should be maintained using vasopressors (e.g. metaraminol) and the heart rate should be maintained between 60 and 80 bpm and in sinus rhythm – 'slow and tight'.
- Neuroaxial blockade should be avoided in patients with severe aortic stenosis. The abrupt and significant fall in SVR can be catastrophic in these patients. That

is because they have a 'fixed' cardiac output. They cannot compensate for any dramatic falls in SVR.
● With the pressure overload, AS patients have concentric LV hypertrophy, which leads to reduced compliance and diastolic dysfunction. They need the 'atrial kick' to fill their LV; therefore, loss of sinus rhythm can be detrimental.

Mitral stenosis

Mitral stenosis patients can proceed with non-cardiac surgery unless symptomatic. The same haemodynamic principles apply: 'slow and tight'.
● Fluid overload can precipitate pulmonary oedema.
● Tachycardia should also be avoided, as it reduces diastolic filling time.
● These patients may be on anticoagulants because of the high risk of thromboembolism.

Aortic regurgitation and mitral regurgitation

This causes a volume overload with eccentric hypertrophy and a dilated, 'baggy' LV. The basic haemodynamic principle is 'fast and loose'.
● Bradycardia should be avoided, as it increases LV end diastolic pressure and can precipitate heart failure.
● These patients tend to tolerate general anaesthesia well, as a reduction in SVR reduces the regurgitant fraction.
● LV function must be assessed preoperatively with echocardiography. If the ejection fraction is low (<30%), then these patients are at high risk for cardiac complications. The risk and benefits should be balanced and surgery is best avoided, if possible.

Prosthetic heart valves

These patients can safely undergo non-cardiac surgery.
   Patients with mechanical heart valves will be on oral anticoagulants. Bridging therapy with intravenous unfractionated heparin is recommended (*see* Table 22.6).
   A high thromboembolic risk is present in:
● mechanical prosthetic heart valves other than bileaflet aortic valve with no risk factors
● biological prosthetic heart valves or mitral valve repair in the last 3 months
● recent thromboembolism (<3 months)
● atrial fibrillation.
   Some examples of high bleeding risk include:
● major vascular procedures
● orthopaedic procedures
● intracranial or spinal neurological procedures
● prostate, bladder or major cancer.

TABLE 22.6 Management of the anticoagulated patient[11]

Low thromboembolic risk/low bleeding risk
Continue oral anticoagulant with INR in therapeutic range
Low thromboembolic risk*/high bleeding risk
Discontinue anticoagulant therapy 48–72 hours before the procedure
Resume within 24 hours of procedure
Therapeutic heparin is usually unnecessary
High thromboembolic risk
Discontinue anticoagulant therapy 5 days before the procedure
Start therapeutic LMWH twice daily or intravenous UFH when the INR falls below 2 (48 hours before surgery)
Give last dose of LMWH 12 hours preop, or continue UFH up to 4–6 hours preop
Resume UFH or LMWH as soon as bleeding status allows; restart oral anticoagulant
Continue LMWH or UFH until INR is therapeutic

INR, international normalised ratio; LMWH, low-molecular-weight heparin; UFH, unfractionated heparin; preop, preoperatively

* Bileaflet mechanical aortic valve replacement with no risk factors (atrial fibrillation, previous thromboembolism, poor LV function, older-generation thrombogenic valves, more than one mechanical valve, mechanical tricuspid valves).

PERMANENT PACEMAKERS AND IMPLANTABLE CARDIOVERTER DEFIBRILLATOR

Preoperative assessment should include a history of the reason for pacing. The pacemaker should be checked unless this has been done within the previous 3 months. Intra-operative principles include the following points.

- Surgical electrocautery interferes with pacemaker and implantable cardioverter defibrillator function.
- Avoid unipolar electrocautery and if used, the ground plate should be as far away from the heart as possible. Bipolar electrocautery is safer.
- Always have an alternative means of pacing available (e.g. external pacing pads).
- Pacemakers with an antitachycardia function or implantable cardioverter defibrillators should be deactivated preoperatively, as they may be triggered by interference from electrocautery. These should be switched back on in recovery before discharge to the ward.

THE HEART TRANSPLANT PATIENT

With improvement in immunosuppression, more of these patients will survive and present for non-cardiac surgery. Special considerations are outlined as follows.

- The transplanted heart has a higher resting heart rate because of absent vagal tone.
- It is preload dependent and therefore the volume status needs to be carefully managed and hypovolaemia avoided.
- Donor hearts do not respond to atropine.
- Donor hearts are prone to early coronary artery disease due to cardiac transplant vasculopathy (32% at 5 years).

- These patients are on immunosuppressants and therefore are at risk of infection.
- Allograft rejection: this can present with new arrhythmias or with symptoms of LV dysfunction (e.g. shortness of breath, paroxysmal nocturnal dyspnoea). Rejection is difficult to diagnose (requires biopsy) and should be treated prior to surgery.

> **Key points**
> - Patients with cardiac disease are at increased risk of morbidity and mortality following non-cardiac surgery.
> - This risk increases as the severity of their cardiac disease and severity of surgery increase. Use scoring systems to quantify risk.
> - They are likely to require additional investigations before surgery.
> - Care must be taken to ensure that they receive the correct cardiac medications before and after surgery.
> - You must know the specific anaesthetic considerations for the individual cardiac conditions.

REFERENCES

1. Devereaux PJ, Yang H, Yusuf S, *et al.* POISE Study Group. Effects of extended-release metoprolol succinate in patients undergoing non-cardiac surgery (POISE trial): a randomized controlled trial. *Lancet.* 2008; **371**(9627): 1839–47.
2. McFalls EO, Ward HB, Moritz TE, *et al.* Predictors and outcomes of perioperative myocardial infarction following elective vascular surgery in patients with documented coronary artery disease: results of the CARP trial. *Eur Heart J.* 2008; **29**(3): 394–401.
3. Tanaka A, Shimada K, Sano T, *et al.* Multiple plaque rupture and C-reactive protein in acute myocardial infarction. *J Am Coll Cardiol.* 2005; **45**(10): 1594–9.
4. Gawande AA, Thomas EJ, Zinner MJ, *et al.* The incidence and nature of surgical adverse events in Colorado and Utah in 1992. *Surgery.* 1999; **126**(1): 66–75.
5. Boersma E, Kertai MD, Schouten O, *et al.* Perioperative cardiovascular mortality in noncardiac surgery: validation of the Lee cardiac risk index. *Am J Med.* 2005; **118**(10): 1134–41.
6. Lee TH, Marcantonio ER, Mangione CM, *et al.* Derivation and prospective validation of a simple index for prediction of cardiac risk of major noncardiac surgery. *Circulation.* 1999; **100**(10): 1043–9.
7. Fleisher LA, Beckman JA, Brown KA, *et al.* American College of Cardiology; American Heart Association Task Force on Practice Guidelines (writing Committee to Revise the 2002 Guidelines on Perioperative Cardiovascular Evaluation for Noncardiac Surgery); American Society of Echocardiography; American Society of Nuclear Cardiology; Heart Rhythm Society; Society of Cardiovascular Anesthesiologists; Society for Cardiovascular Angiography and Interventions; Society for Vascular Medicine and Biology; Society for Vascular Surgery. ACC/AHA 2007 guidelines on perioperative cardiovascular evaluation and care for non-cardiac surgery: a report of the American College of Cardiology/American Heart Association Task Force on Practice Guidelines. *J Am Coll Cardiol.* 2007; **50**(17): e159–241.
8. Le Manach Y, Godet G, Coriat P, *et al.* The impact of postoperative discontinuation or continuation of chronic statin therapy on cardiac outcome after major vascular surgery. *Anesth Analg.* 2007; **104**(6): 1326–33.

9. National Institute for Health and Clinical Excellence. *CardioQ-ODM (Oesophageal Doppler Monitor (MTG3): medical technologies guidance 3*. London: NICE; 2011. www.nice.org.uk/guidance/MTG3

10. Rigg JR, Jamrozik K, Myles PS, *et al*. MASTER Anaethesia Trial Study Group. Epidural anaesthesia and analgesia and outcome of major surgery: a randomised trial. *Lancet*. 2002; **359**(9314): 1276–82.

11. Bonow RO, Carabello BA, Chatterjee K, *et al*. American College of Cardiology/American Heart Association Task Force on Practice Guidelines; Society of Cardiovascular Anesthesiologists; Society for Cardiovascular Angiography and Interventions; Society of Thoracic Surgeons. ACC/AHA 2006 guidelines for the management of patients with valvular heart disease: a report of the American College of Cardiology/American Heart Association Task Force on Practice Guidelines (Writing Committee to Revise the 1998 Guidelines for the Management of Patients with Valvular Heart Disease): developed in collaboration with the Society of Cardiovascular Anesthesiologists: endorsed by the Society of Cardiovascuar Angiography and Interventions and the Society of Thoracic Surgeons. *Circulation*. 2006; **114**(5): e84–231.

CHAPTER 23

The patient with respiratory disease

JUSTIN ROBERTS AND NICK WISELY

Patients with respiratory disease can be divided into patients with an acute illness and those with chronic disease.

Frequently, patients will present for surgery with symptoms of an upper and/or lower respiratory tract infection. Considerable variation exists among anaesthetists regarding their practice in continuing or delaying surgery.

- Those with a fever, cough and chest signs ought to be postponed for up to 4 weeks, because of the risk of exacerbating pulmonary complications.
- Patients, previously well, presenting with simple coryza, without any further symptoms, undergoing minor surgery, can usually be anaesthetised.
- However, some evidence suggests these patients may be at increased risk of developing laryngospasm perioperatively. In practice it is probably best to check with an experienced anaesthetist.

Patients with pre-existing respiratory disease commonly present for surgery. Not infrequently, a patient will have symptoms and signs suggestive of an undiagnosed condition. Respiratory complications occur frequently post-operatively and are associated with significant morbidity and mortality. Those patients with pre-existing respiratory disease are at an increased risk of developing complications. Identifying these patients preoperatively allows optimisation of their therapy and the tailoring of anaesthesia to ameliorate these risks.

Anaesthesia, in particular general anaesthesia, has numerous effects upon the respiratory system. The following are important points:

- reduction in functional residual capacity (FRC)
- FRC encroaches upon closing capacity, resulting in closure of small airways
- increased ventilation–perfusion mismatch
- atelectasis
- volatile induced inhibition of hypoxic pulmonary vasoconstriction
- inhibition of central respiratory drive.

All these factors increase the alveolar-arterial oxygen tension gradient, resulting in hypoxia and impaired CO_2 clearance. These physiological effects are further exacerbated in those with respiratory disease.

Broadly, chronic respiratory conditions are classified into those that limit lung expansion (restrictive disease) and those limiting gas flow (obstructive disease).

- *Restrictive* disease:
  - › intrinsic lung disease such as pulmonary fibrosis
  - › chest wall deformities such as kyphoscoliosis
  - › severe obesity
  - › inspiratory muscle weakness (e.g. muscular dystrophy, myasthenia gravis, spinal cord injury).
- *Obstructive* disease:
  - › asthma
  - › chronic obstructive pulmonary disease
  - › emphysema
  - › bronchiectasis
  - › cystic fibrosis.

Obstructive sleep apnoea, although not typically thought to be an obstructive respiratory condition, causes impaired gas flow during sleep because of loss of pharyngeal tone. This results in a poor sleep pattern, snoring, daytime somnolence and inability to concentrate. This process is exacerbated by anaesthesia.

PREOPERATIVE ASSESSMENT
History

- Determining if a patient's respiratory symptoms are primarily respiratory, cardiac or neuromuscular can be particularly problematic.
- Symptoms suggestive of primary respiratory disease include:
  - › wheeze
  - › cough
  - › sputum production
  - › haemoptysis.
- Respiratory symptoms suggestive of an underlying cardiac condition:
  - › orthopnoea
  - › paroxysmal nocturnal dyspnoea.
- Those with neuromuscular conditions may complain of generalised muscle weakness.
- Is the patient ever short of breath? Is this at rest or upon exertion?
- Exercise tolerance and its limiting factor.
- Cough? Sputum colour? Is this normal for the patient?
- Frequency of respiratory exacerbations in the previous year. Hospital admission? Any critical care admissions?
- Smoking history, both current and past.
- Review regular medications. Does the patient use them regularly as prescribed?
- Oral steroid use in the previous year? Is there a requirement for perioperative supplementation?
- Frequency of use of reliever inhaler therapy?
- Oxygen, nebulisers, continuous positive airway pressure (CPAP) or non-invasive ventilation (NIV) at home?

- The patient's subjective feeling with regard to his or her respiratory function. Is the patient at his or her best?
- Tolerant of non-steroidal anti-inflammatory drugs?

Examination

- All patients should have their oxygen saturations and respiratory rate measured.
- Percussion and auscultation may identify areas of collapse, consolidation, pleural effusions or the presence of pulmonary oedema.
- The presence of wheeze suggests a restriction in gas flow.
- Severe respiratory disease ultimately results in cor pulmonale or right heart failure. This may be evident by dyspnoea at rest, a raised jugular venous pressure and peripheral oedema.

Investigations

- *Peak flow in those with asthma*: this can be compared with the patients 'best' peak flow, if known.
- *Full blood count*: polycythaemia may be evident in chronic hypoxia, leucocytosis in those with active infection.
- *Arterial blood gas*: perform only in those you suspect are retaining CO_2 and in those with severe respiratory disease, particularly if undergoing major surgery.
- *Spirometry*: allows the differentiation of restrictive and obstructive conditions. Irrespective of the diagnosis, an FEV_1 (forced expiratory volume over 1 second) of <1000 mL is likely to limit coughing and sputum clearance post-operatively. Routine spirometry is unnecessary and has not been shown to predict perioperative complications.
- *Chest X-ray*: should be performed in those with an abnormality detected on examination. Those undergoing major thoracic and abdominal surgery with respiratory disease should have a preoperative chest X-ray.
- *Electrocardiograph*: evidence of right ventricular strain or right bundle branch block?
- *Cardiopulmonary exercise testing*: allows quantification of the patient's respiratory limitation.

Optimisation

- Asking patients to stop smoking is likely to be the largest intervention we can do. This is particularly important if the patient is seen many weeks preoperatively. In order to reduce smoking related morbidity, patients should abstain from smoking for 2 months!
- Patients with asthma and chronic obstructive pulmonary disease should have therapy dependent upon its severity as suggested by the British Thoracic Society.
- Patients with poor control or an undiagnosed respiratory problem, which limits their exercise tolerance, presenting for elective surgery should be referred to either their general practitioner or a respiratory physician.
- Asthmatic and chronic obstructive pulmonary disease patients who are wheezy presenting for emergency surgery benefit from nebulised bronchodilator therapy.

- Physiotherapy input for patients with significant sputum load (bronchiectasis and cystic fibrosis) is helpful preoperatively.
- Those with symptoms suggestive of obstructive sleep apnoea should be referred to a physician with an interest in sleep medicine, for investigation and consideration for commencement of CPAP.
- Discuss with the surgical team with regard to incision location (transverse versus midline laparotomy) and the possibility of laparoscopic surgery.

Post-operative care

- Local indications may be in place for critical care admission dependant on patient morbidity and type of surgery.
- Patients with respiratory disease limiting function and in whom major surgery is being undertaken should be admitted to critical care.
- Those requiring preoperative respiratory support (CPAP and NIV) should have a critical care bed booked preoperatively.

THE ANAESTHETIC
General anaesthesia versus regional anaesthesia

- The evidence of superiority for regional anaesthesia over general anaesthesia in all but those with the most severe respiratory disease is lacking. The majority of patients with respiratory conditions tolerate general anaesthesia well.
- Thoracic, major abdominal and laparoscopic surgery in the non-obstetric population on the whole necessitates general anaesthesia.
- Central neuroaxial block (spinal/epidural) can be used for surgery below the umbilicus including lower limb, bladder, peri-anal and prostrate surgery. Regional techniques can be used for surgery above the umbilicus; however, this risks anaesthetising intercostal nerves resulting in respiratory distress. It is important to ensure the patient can lie flat for the period of surgery.
- Local anaesthesia or peripheral nerve blockade are possible for limb, eye and some head and neck surgery. Peripheral nerve blockade is limited by the duration of action of local anaesthesia unless continuous catheter techniques are employed. Care must be taken when anaesthetising nerves in proximity to the phrenic nerve in those with significant respiratory compromise.
- Intravenous regional anaesthesia (such as a Bier's block) is an option for those with limiting respiratory disease undergoing relatively superficial surgery to their limbs.

General anaesthesia

- Avoid drugs that result in the release of histamine in asthmatics or those with a history of bronchospasm if possible (atracurium, mivacurium, and suxamethonium to name a few).
- Ensure those with a salbutamol aerosol inhaler bring it to theatre. The canister, with the aid of a 50 mL syringe can be used to deposit salbutamol in the bronchial tree in the event of bronchospasm while anaesthetised.
- In those with a history of bronchospasm, airway maintenance with a laryngeal mask is beneficial where aspiration isn't a risk. Where intubation is deemed vital, ensure a deep plane of anaesthesia prior to airway instrumentation.

- A spontaneous breathing technique should be used were feasible.
- Ensure adequate humidification of circuits with heat-moisture exchange filters and the use of low-flow anaesthesia.
- When ventilating patients, undertake lung recruitment and utilise positive end-expiratory pressure to maintain lung volume.
- In those ventilated with obstructive lung disorders, the inspiratory:expiratory ratio may need prolongation to ensure adequate exhalation of gases.
- Avoid FiO_2 greater than 80% if possible, as this risks the development of absorption atelectasis intra-operatively.
- Take care when using muscle relaxants, monitor with a nerve stimulator and ensure adequate reversal at the conclusion of surgery.
- In those producing copious sputum, undertake regular tracheal suctioning, particularly prior to extubation.
- Extubate patients sat upright as this increases FRC and aids respiratory mechanics.
- Consideration should be given for extubating patients and commencing CPAP or NIV immediately if the patient uses these preoperatively. This will usually necessitate a critical care admission.

Pain management

- Excellent post-operative analgesia utilising multimodal techniques is key in preventing respiratory complications. This is particularly true for those with abdominal or thoracic incisions. Inadequate analgesia results in:
  › respiratory muscle splinting
  › reduced lung expansion
  › atelectasis and reduced cough effort
  › sputum retention and the development of pneumonia.
- Paracetamol, non-steroidal anti-inflammatory drugs (if appropriate and no contraindication) and tramadol (take care in the elderly) reduce opiate requirements and should be prescribed wherever possible.
- Where spinal anaesthesia is utilised for surgery likely to require post-operative opioids, the addition of diamorphine (300–500 mcg) to the local anaesthetic solution provides analgesia for 12–24 hours.
- Epidural analgesia with low-concentration local anaesthetics, with or without the addition of an opioid, can provide excellent post-operative analgesia in those undergoing open abdominal procedures.
- Trials demonstrating a morbidity and mortality benefit in epidurals are lacking.
- One group that does benefit are those with moderate to severe respiratory disease undergoing a laparotomy. Epidurals have a significant failure rate and those likely to benefit should be cared for in a critical care environment.
- Those undergoing thoracic, non-cardiac surgery benefit from an epidural, epi-pleural or paravertebral catheter technique to provide post-operative analgesia.

Post-operative management

- Patients requiring critical care should be identified preoperatively wherever possible.

- Prescribe oxygen, humidified wherever possible. This is particularly important in those prone to sputum production, as this aids clearance.
- Oxygen ideally should be titrated to SpO_2. A target SpO_2 of 88%–92% is reasonable in those with significant chronic obstructive pulmonary disease or known hypoxia preoperatively. SpO_2 94%–98% for the remainder is sufficient.
- Prescribe nebulised bronchodilator therapy for those with obstructive respiratory conditions.
- Sit patients upright, with the aim of mobilisation as soon as possible.
- A rolled towel to support an abdominal or thoracic incision helps limit pain when coughing.
- Physiotherapy input may help in preventing atelectasis and aid in sputum clearance.
- Careful post-operative fluid balance is vital. Excessive fluid administration increases extravascular lung water, exacerbating any respiratory compromise.
- Ensure venous thromboprophylaxis is prescribed. Use non-pharmaceutical methods (compression stocking and calf compressors) where these are contraindicated.

Key points

- You must decide if the patient has an acute infection that must delay surgery until it has been treated.
- A careful history will be needed if the patient doesn't have a diagnosis for his or her respiratory disease.
- Optimisation of a patient's chronic disease may be vital in order to allow surgery to go ahead and to improve the patient's outcome.
- The surgery may be performed under central-axial or regional anaesthesia. If not, then these can be used to provide post-operative analgesia.
- Physiotherapy and mobilisation are important ways of improving respiratory function after surgery.

CHAPTER 24

Paediatric anaesthesia

NATALIE COOPER AND SIMON MAGUIRE

Anaesthetising children can be stressful and challenging, but it is also rewarding and fun. Children may be anaesthetised as part of an emergency or elective list including adults, or as part of a dedicated paediatric list. Generally, children should be anaesthetised first on the list and in the absence of any other priorities they are anaesthetised in age order. To provide the optimum experience for a child requires a multidisciplinary team, which includes:

- ward nurses
- play therapists
- anaesthetic and recovery staff
- anaesthetists
- surgeons.

Most children will have attended hospital for a play session prior to their admission date in order to prepare them for their anaesthetic and operation. At this time they may also be given age-appropriate information leaflets, such as those produced by the Royal College of Anaesthetists. All children must be seen preoperatively to assess fitness and discuss the anaesthetic plan. This should also help to reduce anxiety and enable a rapport to develop between you, the child and the family.

Paediatric anaesthesia differs from adult anaesthesia in many ways, and this becomes less evident as a child reaches adolescence. Some of the important differences between adults and children are discussed here.

ANATOMY AND PHYSIOLOGY
Airway

- Children's airways are narrower, more compressible and their tongues are larger than in adults. Therefore, it is easy to occlude the airway with your fingers unless you hold only the bony mandible.
- The head is also large in proportion to the body, which can make it difficult to find a neutral point where the airway is open. In preschool children you may need to remove the pillow to achieve this.
- A child's airway is classically described as a funnel shape, with the narrowest

part of the airway at the cricoid ring. An endotracheal tube can cause tissue damage in this area, which may result in tracheal stenosis (discussed later).

- The epiglottis is u-shaped and floppy, which may necessitate the use of a straight blade laryngoscope.
- Children's airways are also more sensitive to instrumentation and they are prone to bradycardia and laryngospasm, especially during light anaesthesia.

Breathing

- A child's respiratory rate is faster than an adult's, decreasing with age. Tidal volumes are approximately 7 mL/kg (*see* Table 24.1 for normal values).

Circulation

- The sympathetic nervous system is immature, so the cardiac output is dependent on heart rate.
- Parasympathetic tone is high and therefore bradycardia is easily precipitated with procedures such as intubation (*see* Table 24.1 for normal values).

TABLE 24.1 Normal physiological parameters[1]

Age (years)	Respiratory rate (breaths per minute)	Heart rate (beats per minute)	Systolic BP
<1	30–40	110–160	70–90
1–2	25–35	100–150	80–95
2–5	25–30	95–140	80–100
5–12	20–25	80–120	90–110
>12	15–20	60–100	100–120

BP, blood pressure

Glucose

- Hypoglycaemia is more common in young children. Maintenance fluids may need to include glucose (as described in the intra-operative section).

Thermoregulation

- Children have a large body surface area:weight ratio, therefore hypothermia occurs rapidly – consider active warming.

BEHAVIOUR AND PSYCHOLOGY[2]

Attending theatre for an operation is a stressful event for a child and for the child's parents. Special measures are taken to prepare the family for anaesthesia, which are generally not seen in adult practice. For example, children over 6 months become distressed when separated from their parents; therefore, parents are allowed to accompany children into the anaesthetic room for induction. The play specialist preparation of children is important for cooperation and distraction and the play specialist will usually be present on induction of anaesthesia.

Children can attend for several anaesthetics during their childhood and so it is important to avoid a traumatic experience. If children are uncooperative it may be beneficial to give them sedative premedication. If a child becomes uncooperative in the anaesthetic room it may be desirable to return them to the ward for sedative premedication prior to continuing. Restraint of a child should be the last resort after considering the urgency of the procedure and obtaining parental agreement.

PHARMACOLOGY

Paediatric drug doses are calculated according to body weight. All children should have an actual weight documented before attending theatre. Approximate weight should only be used in emergencies. Table 24.2 lists the dose per kilogram of commonly used drugs and emergency drugs. It is good practice to calculate the dose of drugs in milligrams and then millilitres of solution for each child prior to induction. This should also be done for emergency drugs such as atropine, suxamethonium and adrenaline, which should be available in the appropriate dilution.

TABLE 24.2 Paediatric doses of commonly used drugs

Drug	Dose	Comment
Propofol	2–4 mg/kg	Titrate to response
Thiopentone	5–7 mg/kg	
Atracurium	0.5 mg/kg	Subsequent doses 1/3 of initial dose
Suxamethonium	1–2 mg/kg	Dilute 100 mg into 10 mL
		4 mg/kg intramuscular dose (neat solution)
Neostigmine/glycopyrrolate	0.02 mL/kg (neat solution)	Dilute one standard ampoule to 5 mL and give 1 mL per 10 kg
Fentanyl	1–2 mcg/kg	
Morphine	0.1 mg/kg	
Paracetamol (PO, PR, IV)	15 mg/kg	Caution: reduce intravenous dose in children less than 10 kg (7.5 mg/kg)
Ibuprofen (PO)	5 mg/kg	
Diclofenac (PR)	1 mg/kg	Ask parental consent first
Ondansetron	0.15 mg/kg	First-line anti-emetic
Dexamethasone	0.15 mg/kg	Second-line anti-emetic
Emergency drugs		
Atropine	10–20 mcg/kg	Dilute in 600 mcg ampoule in 6 mL, 1 mL per 10 kg
Adrenaline	10 mcg/kg	0.1 mL/kg of 1:10 000

PO, oral; PR, rectal; IV, intravenous

PREOPERATIVE

Pre-anaesthetic visit

- The pre-anaesthetic visit is essential for developing a rapport and explaining anaesthesia.

- This should be done in simple non-threatening terms directed at the child as well as the parents.
- Anaesthetic assessment should also include questions regarding:
  > prematurity
  > neonatal problems
  > congenital diseases
  > recent viral illnesses
  > immunisations
  > a cardiorespiratory examination and airway assessment should always be performed.
- Common preoperative problems include upper respiratory tract infections (URTIs) and cardiac murmurs.
- Children can have eight to ten URTIs per year and therefore may attend for anaesthesia with an active or recent URTI.
- These children have a significantly increased risk of a perioperative respiratory complication.
- Children with active illness, pyrexia and purulent secretions should be postponed for 4–6 weeks. Other children should be discussed with the consultant anaesthetist responsible for the list.
- Cardiac murmurs are a common but potentially significant finding, which should be reported to the consultant anaesthetist.

Fasting

Preoperative fasting rules are listed here. Remember that trauma, opiate use and abdominal pathology can prolong gastric emptying.

- Clear fluids: 2 hours
- Breast milk: 4 hours
- Solids: 6 hours

Premedication

- Most children will have local anaesthetic cream such as EMLA (eutectic mixture of local anaesthetics) or topical amethocaine applied to appropriate cannulation sites by the nursing staff.
- Some anaesthetists will prescribe analgesic drugs to be given as premedication, such as paracetamol 15 mg/kg and ibuprofen 5 mg/kg.
- Midazolam can be prescribed orally as a sedative premedicant 30 minutes before induction (0.5 mg/kg; maximum, 20 mg), but it is advisable to discuss this with the consultant anaesthetist first.

INTRA-OPERATIVE

Before the child arrives in the anaesthetic room you should have calculated the doses for all the drugs you may use (including emergency drugs). These drugs should be prepared using antiseptic non-touch technique principles and filter needles. You should also discuss what airway equipment you will need with your anaesthetic assistant and you should have decided on your plan for induction. Even if the consultant has already prepared drugs and equipment, it is good practice to work this out yourself (even if it is just a paper exercise).

Monitoring

- The same monitoring standards apply as for adults. Young children find non-invasive blood pressure measurements distressing, so anaesthetists may choose to delay the first reading until after induction of anaesthesia.

Induction

- The preferred method of induction for children is intravenous. Most children tolerate cannulation well with topical local anaesthesia (EMLA or Ametop) and distraction (e.g. books).
- Induction is usually with titration of propofol and a short-acting opiate. *See* Table 24.2 for doses of commonly used anaesthetic drugs.
- Occasionally a gas induction is performed. There are several methods but a combination of $O_2:N_2O:$sevoflurane 8% is usual. A cooperative child may like to 'blow up the balloon' or 'make the bag whistle', which can ensure large volume breaths. If possible the child is obtunded with $O_2:N_2O$ before sevoflurane is added. It is important to have two trained members of staff, one to maintain the airway while the other is obtaining intravenous access.
- If a rapid sequence induction is indicated cannulation and preoxygenation must be performed prior to induction. Preoxygenation may be aided by play, such as 'blowing up the balloon'. Induction is with thiopentone and suxamethonium, cricoid pressure should be applied by a trained assistant.
- Children have a higher metabolic rate than adults and preoxygenation is not always adequate, so desaturation may occur earlier. It is acceptable to gently ventilate a child via a mask with oxygen (FiO_2 1.0) prior to intubation.

Intravenous access

Intravenous access can be difficult to obtain, especially in infants and toddlers, who often have fat pads on the dorsum of their hands and feet. Common sites for intravenous access include:
- dorsum of the hand
- inner aspect of the wrist
- antecubital fossa (often difficult to find in younger children)
- long saphenous vein (anterior to medial malleolus, this may be attempted blindly in emergencies)
- dorsum of the foot.

Airway

- As discussed earlier, care should be taken not to compress the airway during airway manoeuvres. Oropharyngeal airways may be required, but nasal airways are avoided.
- Oropharyngeal airways should be inserted 'the right way around' because rotation can damage the soft palate.
- Intra-operative airway management is usually with a laryngeal mask airway or endotracheal tube. Laryngeal mask airway sizes are based on weight and are shown in Table 24.3.

TABLE 24.3 Laryngeal mask airway (LMA) sizes based on weight

Weight (kg)	Size of LMA	Maximum air in cuff (mL)
<5	1	4
5–10	1.5	7
10–20	2	10
20–30	2.5	14
30–50	3	20
50–70 (adult)	4	30
>70 (adult)	5	40

Uncuffed endotracheal tubes have traditionally been used for children up to 8–10 years old. This is because the risk of tracheal mucosal damage and subsequent tracheal stenosis is high in prepuberty children at the level of the cricoid. The opinion on this is changing, and some hospitals use specially designed cuffed tubes. Endotracheal tube size is based on age, using the calculation given here (suitable for children over 2 years of age).

Internal diameter = Age/4 + 4.5 mm
Length = Age/2 + 13 cm

- A small leak should be audible following intubation with an uncuffed tube.
- You should have the tube size above and below immediately available.
- You should always auscultate following intubation and after any position changes.
- Endobronchial intubation down either bronchi occurs easily. The tube should be taped to the maxilla. Noting the tube length at the lips or teeth allows any later movement to be corrected immediately.

Laryngoscope blades also differ in paediatric anaesthesia. Straight blade laryngoscopes such as a Magill can be used in infants and small children, these lift the epiglottis directly, rather than sitting in the vallecula. The Macintosh blade (size 2 or 3) can be used for all other children.

Breathing systems and ventilation

- The Ayres T-piece is commonly used for induction of anaesthesia in children less than 20 kg. It is a lightweight, valveless system with low resistance.
- The 500 mL reservoir bag is open-ended and occlusion of this enables controlled ventilation. The use of this system requires practice and complete scavenging of gases is not possible.
- For maintenance of anaesthesia, paediatric circle systems are available. These are suitable for children over 5 kg.
- Paediatric ventilation is often performed with pressure-controlled ventilation, inspiratory pressures 16–20 cmH$_2$O, aiming for tidal volume 8 mL/kg.
- The rate should be adjusted to achieve normocapnia (remember paediatric respiratory rates are higher than adults).

Maintenance and analgesia

- Maintenance is usually achieved with volatile anaesthetic agent, oxygen and nitrous oxide or air. Some anaesthetists use total intravenous anaesthesia; however, this is less common.
- Analgesia should be based on a multimodal approach using drugs and regional analgesia. If not already given preoperatively paracetamol and non-steroidal anti-inflammatory drugs can be given intra-operatively (consent must be taken for suppositories). Opiates may be required (*see* Table 24.2 for doses of commonly used analgesics).
- Infiltration of a local anaesthetic, such as levobupivacaine, should be performed by the surgeons whenever possible. Commonly performed regional anaesthetic techniques include:
  - › caudal analgesia
  - › ilioinguinal block
  - › penile block
  - › transverses abdominus plane block.

Informed consent must be taken for these techniques preoperatively. In the case of caudal analgesia, parents and children must also be warned about post-operative urinary retention and leg weakness. Levobupivacaine is the local anaesthetic of choice for these blocks (maximum, 2 mg/kg).

Fluids

- Intravenous fluid prescription in children can be more complicated.
- In children over 10 kg it is acceptable to use Hartmann's solution in theatre and give 10 mL/kg over the duration of the case.
- However, for prolonged cases and for post-operative maintenance fluid, dextrose and potassium should be included (i.e. 0.45% sodium chloride + 5% dextrose with potassium chloride 10 mmol).

Maintenance fluid is calculated according to the '4-2-1' rule.
- First 10 kg: 4 mL/kg/hour
- Second 10 kg: 2 mL/kg/hour
- Thereafter: 1 mL/kg/hour [e.g. 34 kg = (40 + 20 + 14) = 74 mL/hour]

POST-OPERATIVE

Children should be recovered in an appropriate area with staff trained in paediatric recovery. While in the recovery room any pain and nausea should be assessed and addressed. This can be very difficult in a child who is also distressed because of the unfamiliar environment and people. It can be helpful to ask the parents to come into the recovery room once a child is awake to see if this calms the child.

Pain is assessed using verbal rating scales (e.g. hurts a lot, hurts, hurts a little, doesn't hurt) or faces scales such as the Wong–Baker FACES Pain Rating Scale. Surrogate markers of pain can also be used such as grimacing and positional changes (e.g. guarding). Intravenous morphine may be prescribed for recovery (0.1 mg/kg), but it cannot always be administered on the ward.

Analgesia such as paracetamol and ibuprofen should be prescribed regularly post-operatively with oral opiate doses for breakthrough. Regular analgesia should be taken even when regional anaesthesia is working, so that plasma levels can reach the therapeutic range prior to the block wearing off.

Morphine infusions and patient-controlled analgesia with morphine may be prescribed in appropriate patients if ward nurses are trained to use them (local protocols apply). Children must be mature enough to understand a patient-controlled analgesia, usually over 8 years old, and parents must not use it for the child.

Post-operative nausea and vomiting is less common in children, but it is no less distressing. The current recommendations are to use ondansetron 0.15 mg/kg as first-line rescue treatment. If this has already been given for prophylaxis, dexamethasone 0.15 mg/kg may be given by slow intravenous injection.[3]

REVIEWING CRITICALLY ILL CHILDREN

You may be asked to review a critically unwell child on the ward or in the accident and emergency department. It is important to remember that children can deteriorate quickly and you should call for senior help early. The Advanced Paediatric Life Support cardiac arrest algorithms and guidelines for the management of seizures, choking, anaphylaxis, trauma and burns should be available in all paediatric emergency care areas. The *WETFAG* pneumonic may aid your emergency management while help arrives.

- W: estimated **weight** = (age + 4) × 2
- E: **energy** = 4 J/kg
- T: endotracheal **tube** size = (Age/4) + 4.5 mm
- F: **fluids** = 20 mL/kg (10 mL/kg in trauma)
- A: **adrenaline** = 0.1 mL/kg of 1:10000 solution
- G: **glucose** = 5 mL/kg of 10% dextrose

Key points

- You will find that paediatric anaesthesia can be very different from adult anaesthesia, with new equipment, new staff and new challenges.
- You should prepare individually for each case, making your choice of equipment and drug doses based upon the age and actual weight of the child.
- Never be afraid to seek help or ask for advice.
- Most of all, enjoy anaesthetising children!

REFERENCES

1. Advanced Life Support Group. *Advanced Paediatric Life Support: the practical approach.* 4th ed. London: Blackwell Publishing; 2004.
2. Tan L, Meakin GH. Anaesthesia for the uncooperative child. *Contin Educ Anaesth Crit Care Pain.* 2010; **10**(2): 48–52.
3. Association of Paediatric Anaesthetists of Great Britain and Ireland. *Guidelines on the Prevention of Postoperative Vomiting in Children.* 2009. Accessed at www.apagbi.org.uk/sites/default/files/APA_Guidelines_on_the_Prevention_of_Postoperative_Vomiting_in_Children.pdf

CHAPTER 25

Day case surgery and anaesthesia

KAILASH BHATIA

INTRODUCTION

The definition of day case surgery is not clear. The British definition is a patient who is admitted, has a procedure performed, requires recovery facilities and is discharged the same day and does not stay overnight in the hospital.[1] Other countries accept the definition of less than 24 hours spent by patients in hospital.

In the UK about 65%–70% of elective surgery is done on a day case basis. The Department of Health, as per the National Health Service plan, has set a target of 75% of elective surgery to be performed as day cases. In paediatrics, the European Charter of Children's Rights states: 'Children should be admitted to hospital only if the care they require cannot be equally well provided at home or on a day basis.'[2]

WHY PERFORM DAY SURGERY?

Day surgery has certain advantages pertinent to both patients and the hospital.

Patient benefits

- Decreased time away from home, family and work – definitely suitable not only for the young patients but also for those at extremes of age, for it decreases the separation from the familiar home environment
- Less stress and emotional disturbance
- Reduced risk of infection, as shorter hospital stay

Hospital benefits

- Less dependence on availability of hospital beds
- More efficient use of operating rooms
- Less preoperative testing and post-operative medication
- Greater flexibility in scheduling operations
- Lower staffing requirements
- Lower overall procedure costs for the hospital

SELECTION CRITERIA FOR DAY SURGERY

Accurate selection of both the procedures and patients is the key to safe and effective day case surgery. Criteria can be divided into:

- social
- surgical
- medical.

Social criteria

- The patient must be willing to undergo surgery on a day case basis.
- The patient must have a responsible adult to escort him or her home by car or taxi and remain with him or her for the first 24 hours after surgery.
- The patient must live within 1 hour from the hospital.
- The patient should have easy access to a telephone.
- The patient's home situation should be compatible with post-operative care, with satisfactory standards of heating and lighting, together with adequate kitchen, bathroom and toilet facilities.
- The patient should have general practitioner backup available.

Surgical criteria

The surgery should be predictable and should not last longer than 120 minutes, although this is no longer a strict criterion. Even complex surgery such as laparoscopic cholecystectomy and Nissan's fundoplication are being done on a day case basis.

The surgery should not involve major blood loss, major fluid shifts or require large amounts of opioids.

Medical criteria

- ASA 1 and 2 (American Society of Anesthesiologists Classification 1 and 2) patients.
- Medically stable ASA 3 (American Society of Anesthesiologists Classification 3) patients.
- There is no age limit to day case surgery. Selection should be based on functional limitation rather than just the presence of disease.

CONTRAINDICATIONS TO DAY SURGERY

With improving anaesthetic techniques and with major advances in minimal access surgery, patients with complex medical conditions can undergo day case surgery. However, there are groups of patients who would be at increased risk of complications post-operatively and would not be suitable for day case anaesthesia. These are:

- symptomatic life-threatening conditions (e.g. angina, uncontrolled diabetes, epilepsy, asthma, congestive cardiac failure)
- myocardial infarction within the last 3 months
- morbid obesity with cardiovascular or respiratory complications
- the lack of a responsible adult at home to take care of the patient or unfavourable social conditions
- open peritoneal surgery associated with major blood loss, fluid shifts or severe pain

- ex–premature babies less than 60 weeks' post-conceptual age who are at risk of apnoeas.

ASSESSMENT AND PREOPERATIVE INVESTIGATIONS

Assessment is usually nurse led on an outpatient basis with input from anaesthetists and frequently consists of questionnaires and protocols. Early assessment allows time for specialist referral, the necessary investigations and corrective action to be taken without delaying surgery. *See* Chapter 4 for the relevant investigations and their indications.

PREPARING FOR DAY SURGERY

After preoperative assessment, patients agree a date for their surgery. Patients are given specific information via leaflets about the procedure. They need to be told where and when to come. In day case units the admissions are usually staggered. Full written information about what to bring to the hospital, which medications to take, the patient's escort and about fasting (6 hours for solids and a 2-hour period for clear liquids) should be provided. Also, the patients are informed of the people they will meet when they come to the unit.

The ideal model is a self-contained day surgery unit in a hospital, with its own admission suite, wards, theatre and recovery area, together with administrative facilities.[3] Another possibility is a day case ward with patients going to the main operating theatre where lists may be made up entirely of day cases. Every day case suite must have facilities to admit the patient in hospital if required. Close cooperation between the general practitioners, surgeons, anaesthetists, theatre staff, nurses and the patient is vital to an efficient day case unit.

The patient arrives at the admission suite and is seen by a senior nurse and admitted to the ward. The anaesthetist and the surgeon assess the patient, explaining to the patient the procedure he or she is about to undergo. The anaesthetist should focus on the clinical history, allergies and airway. For children and needle-phobic patients, Ametop or EMLA (eutectic mixture of local anaesthetics) creams are popular. Nonsteroidal anti-inflammatory drugs (NSAIDs) given orally 30 minutes before surgery achieve peak levels at the end of procedure and are a useful adjunct to anaesthesia.

ANAESTHETIC CONSIDERATIONS

The patient usually walks into the anaesthetic room or is wheeled in on a trolley. Intravenous access is established and the Association of Anaesthetists of Great Britain and Ireland minimum standards of monitoring are used perioperatively (*see* Chapter 5). The aim is to provide rapid and safe anaesthetic conditions for surgical procedures with a rapid and predictable recovery. You want to avoid pain and post-operative nausea and vomiting (PONV). Anaesthetic options that are available include:

- general anaesthesia
- regional anaesthesia
- sedation
- local anaesthesia
- a combination of these options.

GENERAL ANAESTHESIA

It remains a popular choice for most day case surgery especially with the availability of modern anaesthetic agents with excellent recovery profiles.

Induction agent

Propofol remains the induction agent of choice. It has a quick onset and a favourable recovery profile. In children, inhalational induction with sevoflurane (if unable to secure intravenous access) is an acceptable alternative.

Airway

The laryngeal mask is a clear favourite because it avoids intubation (including muscle relaxants and reversal), is easy to place and is tolerated well at lighter levels of anaesthesia. Tracheal intubation is an acceptable option provided short- or intermediate-acting muscle relaxants are used (e.g. mivacurium). Suxamethonium should be avoided because of its side effect profile, especially muscle aches.

Analgesia

A balanced analgesic regime is vital. Low doses of opioids (e.g. incremental doses of fentanyl) in combination with NSAIDs (or cyclo-oxygenase 2 inhibitors) and local anaesthetic agents are generally adequate for surgery. Morphine is an unpopular option because it increases rates of sedation and levels of PONV.

Maintenance of anaesthesia

Sevoflurane or isoflurane with spontaneous respiration using a mixture of oxygen and air mixture via a laryngeal mask airway are the usual. Nitrous oxide is used in children as a carrier gas (it reduces the minimum alveolar concentration of inhalational agents) but in adults it's avoided for its association with PONV. Desflurane is an attractive option because of its quick recovery profile, especially in obese patients. In patients at high risk of PONV, total intravenous anaesthesia with propofol can be used for both induction and maintenance, as it has anti-emetic properties.

Intravenous fluids

Hydration with a litre of crystalloid has been shown to reduce drowsiness and PONV during the recovery period and is recommended for all day surgery patients who have a general anaesthetic.

Anti-emetics

There should be a PONV risk assessment for every patient undergoing day surgery. This and the treatment options can be found in Chapter 17.

REGIONAL ANAESTHESIA

Appropriate timing and planning are important if regional anaesthesia is to be successfully used for day case surgery. The advantages of using regional anaesthesia are good post-operative pain relief (opioid-free anaesthesia) with less PONV.

Spinal anaesthesia

This could be used for any lower limb, urological or inguinal surgery especially in patients with chronic obstructive pulmonary disease or morbid obesity. It should be performed early on the list to allow maximum time for it to wear off. Low doses of bupivacaine (5 mg) are used along with a small amount of intrathecal fentanyl. Disadvantages include prolonged motor block, urinary retention and headache, all of which could result in an overnight stay. Caudal and epidurals are not popular choices for they limit mobility and large volumes of local anaesthetic are required.

Peripheral nerve blocks

Any peripheral block can be used to facilitate day case surgery as long as it does not limit mobility. Lower concentrations (0.25% bupivacaine) should be used to provide analgesia. They could be used alone (*see* Chapter 27), or in combination with a general anaesthetic or with some sedation. Plexus blocks (brachial plexus) are popular choices for upper limb surgery. Patients will require specific instructions on care of the anaesthetised limb so as to avoid inadvertent damage following hospital discharge.

SEDATION

Midazolam sedation in titrated doses (e.g. endoscopy) can be used for day case patients. A target-controlled infusion of propofol can also be used.

POST-OPERATIVE CONSIDERATIONS

After the procedure, patients are transferred to a recovery room. Adequate post-operative analgesia for recovery should be prescribed – this commonly involves incremental doses of fentanyl, NSAIDs and paracetamol (if not already given in theatre). Rescue anti-emetics also need to be prescribed. You may have to prescribe the prescription to take home. These consist of simple analgesics such as paracetamol, codeine and NSAIDs. If NSAIDs are not tolerated then tramadol is an acceptable alternative.

The usual criteria are used for discharge from recovery (*see* Chapter 12). Some centres use specific systematic approach and scoring criteria before patients are discharged from the recovery to the ward bay. A senior nurse ensures that all the following criteria listed are met before the patient is discharged from the hospital and day case suite.

CRITERIA FOR DISCHARGE FOLLOWING DAY SURGERY

- The patient must be oriented in time, place and person.
- The patient must have stable observations within predetermined limits.
- No surgical complications.
- Acceptable pain control and absent or minimal nausea and vomiting.
- If the patient has received a spinal anaesthesia, then he or she must have return of full motor power.
- The patient must eat, drink and have passed urine.
- The intravenous cannula must be removed and the wound must be dry.
- The patient should be able to dress and be mobile.
- A responsible adult must take the patient home and provide care for the next 24 hours.
- The patient should have adequate analgesia prescribed and available.

- The patient requires clear instructions to avoid alcohol, driving and using machinery for the next 24–48 hours.
- The patient should have the appropriate information including hospital telephone numbers in case of an emergency, any follow-up that is required and a general practitioner letter.

Key points

- Meticulous planning and organisation is required for successful and efficient day case surgery.
- Strict criteria have to be met before day surgery is performed and before the patient is discharged from the hospital.
- Preoperative investigations are not necessary for fit and well patients.
- Propofol is the most popular anaesthetic agent and the laryngeal mask airway is the most common airway device used.
- Multimodal analgesic regimens using a combination of local anaesthesia, NSAIDs and opioids should be used for pain management.
- Ensure adequate hydration and PONV risk assessment for all patients undergoing day surgery.
- Pain, PONV and bleeding after surgery are the most common factors leading to unanticipated admission after day surgery.

REFERENCES

1. Department of Health. *The NHS Plan: a plan for investment, a plan for reform.* London: Department of Health; 2000.
2. Verma R, Alladi R, Jackson I, *et al.* Day case and short stay surgery: 2. *Anaesthesia.* 2011; **66**: 417–34.
3. Royal College of Anaesthetists. *Guidance on the Provision of Anaesthetic Services.* London: Royal College of Anaesthetists; 2009.

CHAPTER 26

Transferring the anaesthetised patient

MATTHEW STAGG AND PAUL DEAN

However experienced the anaesthetist, transferring a patient is a daunting task. Anaesthetists often find themselves transferring patients both within the hospital and between hospitals. These patients are often very sick, the vast majority are intubated and ventilated and they are usually being moved to more specialised areas for expert care such as neurosurgery or paediatrics. Transferring patients, even a short distance, can be challenging and potentially dangerous. For this reason, care and due attention must be taken and all eventualities planned for prior to embarking on transfer. Fortunately, in spite of all the dangers, probably because we are very aware of the risks, most transfers are completed without difficulty.

THE DECISION TO TRANSFER

The decision to transfer must be based on the need for specific clinical intervention versus the risks of the associated transfer. Factors influencing this decision include:

- the specific nature of the injury, including those where time to treatment is vital
- the likely success of the treatment
- the presence of individual patient co-morbidities
- the risks associated with the transfer
- the personal beliefs and wishes of the patient.

Once it is decided to transfer a patient, this must be clearly documented in the clinical notes, stating the time and date the decision was made, whether the decision was discussed with other medical staff, the family and why it was occurring.

Wherever possible, the transfer of a patient from one place of safety to another must be carried out in an organised, timely fashion, with optimisation, stabilisation and resuscitation of the patient's condition occurring well in advance. This process may take several hours after the initial decision has been made.

Other patient transfers are extremely time dependent (e.g. a ruptured abdominal aortic aneurysm or an extradural haematoma). Here time delays are a greater risk to the patient. In such circumstances, senior support is vital.

PLANNING A TRANSFER

When the decision is made to transfer a patient between hospitals, several important handovers must occur.

- First, a medical team at the destination hospital must agree to take over the care of the patient.
- Second, bed managers need to be informed both at transferring and receiving hospitals in order to confirm a bed is available.
- Third, a critical care bed must be arranged. This is frequently done 'consultant to consultant'.

In most areas of the UK, regional networks will coordinate, where critical care beds are available. Where more specialised tertiary services are required (e.g. extracorporeal membrane oxygenation), this is done nationally. Standardised protocols, documentation and equipment are usually present within networks. This also provides an audit trail to help improve the service.

Throughout the UK there are a limited number of retrieval teams (based mainly in the field of paediatric critical care) that will provide a specialised team to collect the patient.

Most transfers in the UK occur by road; however, there are increasing numbers of transfers occurring by rotary or fixed-wing aircraft, either because of the distance, the speed at which the patient needs to be transferred or because the casualty is inaccessible by road. Transferring patients by this method poses additional hazards (variable pressures, expanding air-filled spaces, temperature changes) that require specialist training and are beyond the scope of this book.

THE TRANSFER

Personnel

The Association of Anaesthetists of Great Britain and Ireland (AAGBI) advise that patients who are unlikely to need airway or ventilator support, patients for whom cardiopulmonary resuscitation would be inappropriate, patients being transferred for acute definitive management for whom anaesthesia support will not affect their outcome and patients not likely to require specialist drugs do not need the presence of an anaesthetist.[1] Ultimately, it is the responsibility of the senior clinicians arranging the transfer, in discussion with their respective specialist teams to choose the most appropriate member of medical staff to accompany the patient.

- A critically ill patient should be accompanied by a minimum of two carers (anaesthetist and operating department practitioner or nurse).[1]
- The doctor transferring the patient must be appropriately experienced, not only in transferring critically ill patients but also in the management of any complications that may arise on the way.
- Ideally, where an anaesthetist is required he or she should be experienced both in hospital and transfer medicine and have attended at least one or more of the prominent transfer courses available throughout the UK.
- A 'live' inter-hospital transfer is often not the time to be concentrating on the education of those less experienced in the field; however, pre-transfer teaching and as much experience in intra-hospital transferring, under the supervision of

an experienced clinician, is highly recommended for those less confident to gain the skills required.

- A trained assistant is required to accompany the doctor. Going on a transfer alone is not acceptable. The assistants should again be appropriately trained in all the equipment and drugs that may need to be utilised and have experience in assisting in the management of airways and critically ill patients.
- Most trusts have appropriate policies and guidance stating who should be going on transfers.

Monitoring, equipment and drugs

The close observation and monitoring of an anaesthetised patient is vital and this is made even more apparent on a transfer. Patients should receive the same standard of physiological monitoring during transfer as if they were still on an ICU.[2] Familiarity with all equipment that may be used is paramount and first-time use on a transfer is not appropriate. The minimum standard of monitoring for the transfer includes:

- blood pressure monitoring (usually invasive)
- continuous electrocardiograph
- SpO_2
- temperature
- if intubated, end-tidal carbon dioxide monitoring.

Appropriate venous access must be obtained; the clinical scenario dictating whether this is central multi-lumen intravenous catheters or two large-bore peripherally located cannulae. Up-to-date blood results must be available, as well as all radiological investigations.

If your patient is ventilated you must be fully trained to use the transfer ventilator. Experience and knowledge of commonly used transfer ventilators (e.g. Dräger Oxylog®) is mandatory. It must be set up appropriately.

- Disconnection, high pressure and low oxygen alarms must be active and set to appropriate levels with both audible and visual alarms that can be heard above the noise and vibration of an ambulance.
- Most ventilators have the ability to supply positive end-expiratory pressure, variable inspired oxygen concentration, an ability to change the inspiratory: expiratory ratio, as well as adjust the respiratory rate and tidal volume.
- More modern ventilators now have the additional bonus of delivering ventilation through pressure-controlled modes, pressure support modes or even just continuous positive airway pressure.

All patients being transferred should have a chest X-ray to confirm correct endotracheal tube placement and exclude pneumothorax from central line placement.

Running out of oxygen on a transfer is extremely dangerous and may result in a fatality. Make sure that you are aware of exactly how much oxygen is present in the cylinders and how long that supply will last based on the flow rates that are set for the patient. Compare this with the expected distance and time that it will need to be available for and make sure that plenty is spare (i.e. double the amount!). Tables for reference can be found in various publications, including the *Oxford Handbook of Anaesthesia*.[3]

Many trusts or departments now have a specific transfer trolley, with storage space for cylinders, a transfer ventilator, suction equipment and syringe drivers. Ensure it is compatible with the model of ambulance being sent to transfer the patient.

Most emergency departments, critical care units and theatres have pre-packaged transfer bags complete with all the kit required for a transfer. The same basic equipment should be present in all of them.

- Basic airway management equipment:
  - ❭ oropharyngeal airways
  - ❭ endotracheal tubes
  - ❭ spare laryngoscopes including batteries
  - ❭ alternative laryngoscopy blades
  - ❭ bougie
  - ❭ stethoscopes
  - ❭ self-inflating ventilation bag
  - ❭ suction devices.
- Cardiovascular equipment:
  - ❭ replacement cannulae
  - ❭ needles and syringes
  - ❭ fluids and giving sets.
- Emergency drugs:
  - ❭ adrenaline, atropine and amiodarone
  - ❭ metaraminol or noradrenaline drawn up
  - ❭ any other drugs you think that you may require
  - ❭ the dates must be checked to guarantee that these drugs will still be effective.
- Always ensure that all syringe pumps being used are fully charged and that at least one spare syringe driver is taken.

THE AMBULANCE

It is most likely that the ambulance will be requested from the local ambulance service. A 'Type B' variety will only have 12 V electric sockets, oxygen supply with limited monitoring and other equipment. Therefore, it is vital that the ample oxygen cylinders are available and that all electrical equipment is fully charged and will last for the length of the transfer. Spare batteries for all other equipment must be carried.

The Association of Anaesthetists of Great Britain and Ireland (AAGBI) guidelines on transferring a patient state that the ambulance should have means of securing the trolley with access to all sides and with the fixation capable of withstanding at least 10 G in all directions.[1]

Also, acknowledge that gravity-dependent drips are unreliable in this degree of motion and therefore syringe drivers should be employed wherever possible.

PRACTICAL HINTS

- Transferring patients makes them cold. Unless this is your intention, use all appropriate measures to keep them warm. Don't forget, you can ask to have the heat turned up in the back of the ambulance.
- Use tape! Make sure all cannulae, transducers and anything attached to the patient are secured. It is useful to secure pressure transducers to the patient's upper arms or chest wall.

- Whilst it is exciting to be speeding through towns with blue lights flashing and sirens sounding, it is rarely necessary to be travelling at excessive speed. Equipment can become projectiles, and it can mean nausea for you, and cardiovascular instability for your patient.
- High visibility and, where necessary, warm clothing, money, food and a mobile phone are a must. No one can guarantee exactly how long you will be away from the hospital and being cold and hungry in an unknown location with no ability to even buy a cup of tea is very demoralising.
- Knowing the contact numbers of colleagues and the hospital you are transferring to is vital in case help or advice is needed.
- Make sure that you or someone in your transfer party knows exactly where you are going.
- As a mark of professional courtesy, inform the receiving unit just as you are leaving and give your expected time of arrival so they can be prepared.
- Ensure that all of the patient's notes are complete and copied if required, and that the patient's belongings are together for transfer or given to a relative to look after.
- Having relatives on a transfer is unwise and usually impossible. Depending on the physical condition of the patient, the age and the length of transfer having a single relative may be acceptable, but this must be taken on a case-by-case basis.
- Make certain that all of the equipment taken with you is returned to the correct site.

Remember, as with so much in medicine, there is no substitute for practice and experience, and success and safety is so often produced through appropriate and thorough preparation. The same wise words can be applied to critically ill patient transfer, whatever the situation.

Key points
- Any patient who requires you to transfer them will be sick and potentially unstable. Only people who are qualified to do it should transfer the patient.
- Preparation is the key. You have to recreate intensive care in an ambulance.
- Check all your equipment and drugs before you go and ensure that you have spares and backups.
- Ensure that you know where you are going and that they are expecting you at that time. You must take the notes and investigations with you.
- Make sure that you have the transport or the money to get yourself and your equipment home.

REFERENCES

1. Association of Anaesthetists of Great Britain and Ireland. *Interhospital Transfer.* London: AAGBI; 2009.
2. Association of Anaesthetists of Great Britain and Ireland. *Recommendations for the Safe Transfer of Patients with Brain Injury.* London: AAGBI; 2006.
3. Allman K, Wilson I. *Oxford Handbook of Anaesthesia.* 2nd ed. New York, NY: Oxford University Press; 2007. p. 855.

CHAPTER 27

Regional anaesthesia

ZARA TOWNLEY

Regional anaesthesia involves, in its simplest terms, injecting local anaesthetic around a nerve to provide analgesia or anaesthesia to the area that that nerve supplies. This may be done centrally, where the nerves leave the spinal cord (e.g. spinals or epidurals), or peripherally, where the individual nerves can be targeted (e.g. a femoral nerve block).

Ultrasound allows visualisation of the target, and as success rates are improving, regional anaesthesia is increasing in popularity.

However, before you even get your hands on a Tuohy needle or a nerve stimulator there are a few general points that need to be covered in preparation for a regional technique.

DOES YOUR PATIENT NEED REGIONAL ANAESTHESIA?

There are some advantages to regional techniques, as outlined here.

A safe alternative to general anaesthesia

- For those patients who may be high risk, use of a sole regional technique may be preferable (e.g. a patient with severe chronic obstructive pulmonary disease).
- Some patients may prefer to be awake and avoid the side effects of a general anaesthetic (e.g. a woman having an elective caesarean section).

The provision of peri- and post-operative analgesia

- Regional techniques can provide excellent pain relief post-operatively and therefore avoid the use of strong opiates.
- This may provide faster recovery and earlier discharge.

Other possible benefits

- There has been a lot of interest over the years in the possibility of regional anaesthesia reducing stress responses, improving morbidity and mortality and, more recently, reducing cancer recurrence, but so far the evidence has been equivocal.

SO WHY DON'T ALL OF OUR PATIENTS HAVE REGIONAL ANAESTHESIA?

Despite the advantages stated, there would be patients who are not suitable for a regional technique:

- someone with a clotting abnormality
- those who do not want to be awake during their operation or who do not consent
- those where the surgery being performed doesn't lend itself to a regional technique (e.g. a total laryngectomy).

Sometimes the combination of a general anaesthetic with a regional technique is the best option. Each patient is individual and has different needs depending on the patient and his or her surgery. Therefore, the decision to use regional anaesthesia is one that comes with experience, so don't expect to get it right on day one – have a look at your list for the day and discuss the patients with your consultant. Your consultant will be able to advise you on whether he or she would consider using a regional technique for any of the patients on the list. This will help you when you go to see your patients preoperatively.

THE PREOPERATIVE VISIT

The preoperative visit should include the following.

- A general anaesthetic assessment – as for a general anaesthetic, even if regional is being considered as the sole technique. A general anaesthetic is your plan B.
- Exclusion of absolute contraindications:
  › allergy to local anaesthetic agents
  › local infection or trauma at the needle insertion site
  › patient refusal.
- Identification of relative contraindications:
  › sepsis
  › coagulation disorder or anticoagulant therapy
  › co-morbidities (e.g. aortic stenosis and spinals)
  › anatomical anomalies
  › hypovolaemia
  › raised intracranial pressure.
- An explanation of the technique and benefits.
- An explanation of the risks (see *Complications*).

If you aren't familiar with all of the risks and benefits of all the regional techniques your consultant must take the consent. It is important to document discussions with patients regarding risks and consent on the anaesthetic form. For more information, the Royal College of Anaesthetists website provides patient information leaflets that outline the risk of nerve damage from spinal, epidural and regional anaesthesia.[1]

IN THE ANAESTHETIC ROOM

At the start of your training it is important that you know how to prepare yourself, your consultant and the patient for the technique once they have arrived in the anaesthetic room. If this has already been done for you by your operating department practitioner or anaesthetic nurse you must check it, as it is your responsibility.

Monitoring

All patients who have a regional anaesthetic should have the same minimum monitoring as those about to have a general anaesthetic. This should commence prior to the start of the block and be recorded regularly.

Resuscitation equipment

This must be in working order and readily available. This includes accessibility to Intralipid, a lipid emulsion that is included in the Association of Anaesthetists of Great Britain and Ireland guidelines for the management of local anaesthetic toxicity.[2]

Intravenous access

All patients should have intravenous access established prior to commencement of any regional technique.

Equipment

- Appropriate needles plus or minus catheters for the block
- Sterile field
- Appropriate cleaning solution
- Local anaesthetic, both for skin infiltration and for the block
- Nerve stimulator
- Ultrasound machine
- Appropriate dressings

To begin with, you will be observing these procedures and it is important that you use this time to watch the consultant performing the procedure. You will notice that each consultant will have his or her own technique, from drawing up the drugs, to cleaning the skin, to performing the actual procedure. The key is to take all of these tips on board and when you get to perform the procedure yourself you will apply what you have learned and under guidance eventually refine your technique.

LOCAL ANAESTHETICS

You may use high volumes of local anaesthetic and it is important to know which local anaesthetic to choose and how much it is safe to give.

TABLE 27.1 Comparison of commonly used local anaesthetics

	Lignocaine	Bupivacaine	L-bupivacaine	Ropivacaine
pKa value	7.9	8.1	8.1	8.07
Protein binding (%)	75	95	97	94
Potency	1	4	4	4
Maximum dose (mg/kg)	3 (6 with adrenaline)	2	2.5	3
Onset (minutes)	5–15	10–20	<15	10–15
Duration	Medium	Long	Long	Long

The pharmacology of each local anaesthetic is related to its duration of action, speed of onset and toxicity, but this is something to read up on for the Fellowship of the Royal College of Anaesthetists exam. Table 27.1 describes the properties of the most common local anaesthetics and their maximum dose. These factors will influence the choice of local for each regional block and often they are used in combination to get the best of both worlds!

NEUROTOXICITY

The initial neurological manifestation of toxicity is often subtle and can easily be missed if you are not paying attention. The patient may become garrulous or he or she may suddenly go quiet. The key is to keep talking to your patient!

The other symptoms include:

- perioral tingling
- tinnitus
- nystagmus
- dizziness
- restlessness
- tremor
- convulsions
- coma.

CARDIOTOXICITY

These effects usually come after the first signs of neurotoxicity but be warned, the only sign of toxicity may be cardiorespiratory arrest! The signs include:

- myocardial depression with hypotension
- cardiac arrhythmias
- ventricular arrest.

Bupivacaine has a narrower safety margin and takes a long time to dissociate from the myocardium, often requiring prolonged cardiopulmonary resuscitation. For this reason some of the newer agents – for example, L-bupivacaine (an enantomer of bupivacaine) and ropivacaine – are being increasingly used, especially when larger volumes are required (e.g. lower limb nerve blocks).

MANAGEMENT OF LOCAL ANAESTHETIC TOXICITY

Local anaesthetic toxicity has been notoriously hard to treat and in the case of cardiac arrest the outcomes were poor. With the advent of Intralipid, however, there is a growing number of cases reporting that it is very useful in the treatment of local anaesthetic toxicity. The Association of Anaesthetists has recently updated its guidelines on the treatment of local anaesthetic toxicity and Intralipid.[2]

The most important step is to avoid toxicity in the first place.

- Know your maximum safe doses and keep below them.
- Repeatedly aspirate during injection of local anaesthetic.
- If you're using ultrasound, stop injecting if you can't see it on the screen.
- Talk to your patient throughout the procedure.

SPINAL ANAESTHESIA

Indications

- Spinal anaesthesia can be used for a wide variety of surgical procedures to the lower body below the umbilicus (e.g. caesarean section, total hip replacement).

Anatomy

- The technique involves injecting a small amount of local anaesthetic into the cerebrospinal fluid at the lumbar level.
- The spinal cord ends at L1/L2 in adults but the dura ends at S2; therefore, the injection is usually performed at the L3–4, L4–5 or L5–S1 interspaces.
- A line joining both iliac crests (Tuffier's line) passes across the spine of L4 and is the landmark most often used to locate the L3/4 interspace.

Equipment

- The Sprotte or Whitacre spinal needles and introducers are designed to reduce the incidence of post-dural puncture headache. The gauge varies from 22 to 29 G; the larger needles are easier to use but increase the risk of headache.
- The local anaesthetic most commonly used for spinals is 0.5% 'heavy' bupivacaine. The 'heavy' bit relates to the fact that glucose makes the solution heavier than cerebrospinal fluid and therefore it will sink under gravity. Positioning the patient can move the local anaesthetic within the cerebrospinal fluid (e.g. keeping the patient in the sitting position for a saddle block for perineal surgery).
- Adjuncts such as opiates, which alter the effect of the block. The dose of each of these will vary depending on what surgical procedure the anaesthetic is for.

Technique

As discussed earlier, preparation is the key to success with any regional technique. Before positioning, it is important that you have secured venous access with a wide-bore cannula and full monitoring is applied.

The patient is then positioned either in the lateral or the sitting position. The choice of position is usually a personal preference but sometimes the patient dictates it (e.g. patients with fractured neck of femurs).

At this point it may be worth palpating the patient's back to identify the appropriate space before scrubbing up.

Strict asepsis is required for this procedure and it is expected that you will scrub up, using gown, gloves, hat and mask. A sterile pre-filled pack is usually available and your anaesthetic assistant will open this for you and pass any other bits of equipment that you need, including your choice of spinal needle.

Spinals are a tactile as well as a visual procedure and it is important to get the feel as your needle moves through the different layers and the final 'give' as you pass through the ligamentum flavum into the dura.

Once the procedure is finished, it is then vital to monitor the patient regularly, as the sympathetic block causes marked vasodilatation with a reduction in cardiac output and blood pressure. This effect is more marked if the patient is dry, so intravenous fluids must be running prior to the procedure. They may also become bradycardic if the block goes very high.

It is also important to position the patient appropriately before the block 'fixes'. This is usually supine but may be lateral, with the operative side down.

The block must be tested prior to commencing surgery as these patients are in most cases not having a general anaesthetic. Sensory blockade is tested most commonly with ethyl chloride spray but light touch is more reliable. However, it is important that you know your dermatomes! Testing for lack of function tests motor block.

Once the block is effective and the patient is stable then the patient can be transferred into the theatre for surgery. The patient may be given sedation at this point and full monitoring is continued throughout the procedure. The patient may require oxygen.

Complications
- Immediate:
  > hypotension
  > high block.
- Delayed:
  > post-dural puncture headache
  > urinary retention
  > haematoma formation
  > infection
  > direct nerve damage
  > cord ischaemia.

EPIDURAL ANAESTHESIA
As a new starter in anaesthesia you probably won't be performing epidurals and it may be well into your training before you do your first one. You will usually do lumbar epidurals first and then, once you have mastered the technique, progress to thoracic ones.

They are a very important skill to learn. They often form an important part of the anaesthetic plan for major thoraco-abdominal surgery especially in the high-risk patient. Equally as important is the obstetric epidural.

Indications
- In addition to general anaesthesia to reduce perioperative opiates
- As a sole anaesthetic technique (e.g. for caesarean section)
- As a sole analgesic technique (e.g. for labour or fractured ribs)
- For post-operative pain relief, either as part of the anaesthetic plan or as a rescue technique
- In treatment of chronic pain

Anatomy
- An epidural involves putting local anaesthetic into the extradural space.
- This space is reached by passing the needle posteriorly through skin, subcutaneous tissue, spinous ligaments and then the ligamentum flavum.
- It involves using much larger volumes of local anaesthetic and in most cases placement of a catheter into that space.
- The midline approach is most commonly used but the space can also be approached from the paramedian.

To begin the procedure it is important to identify the correct interspace. Where you go will depend on what the epidural is for and how high you need the block to go (e.g. T10–11 for lower abdominal procedures, T8–9 for upper abdominal procedures).

Equipment

Tuohy needles are used for epidurals – they have a blunt tip, which is designed to reduce the risk of dural puncture and is curved to guide catheter direction. The most common sizes used are 16 and 18 G. The needles have a stiletto, which is removed once the needle is inserted into the interspinous ligament. The needles usually come in a pack with the catheter, bacterial filter and loss-of-resistance syringe.

Technique

The preparation for the procedure is identical to that for a spinal injection including monitoring, intravenous access, positioning and strict asepsis.

Go through the epidural kit making sure nothing is missing and it is all set up ready to use. You will need local anaesthetic for skin infiltration and normal saline for flushing the catheter and finding the epidural space.

After preparation of the injection site and infiltration of your local anaesthetic (be generous here, as the procedure can be painful) you are ready to start the procedure.

The 'loss of resistance' technique is used for epidural insertion.

- The ligamentum flavum is a very dense ligament through which it is almost impossible to inject, but on reaching the epidural space there is negative pressure, which will make it very easy to inject through the syringe.
- Traditionally air was used to locate the space but now normal saline is mostly used to avoid the risk of air embolus.
- Everyone does this slightly differently but the key is to take your time and make sure that your driving pressure on the syringe is always through the plunger so that when you do enter the epidural space only the plunger moves in and not the needle!
- Once you have located the space you can then feed your catheter through the needle. Ensure that you feed plenty of catheter in, so that when you pull your needle out over your catheter you don't risk dislodging the catheter out of the space.
- The catheter is then generally withdrawn to leave 4–6 cm in the space. It is important to note the depth of the space before you withdraw the needle so you know what length the catheter should be at the skin.
- Once the catheter is in place there are a few checks you can do to reassure yourself that you are in the right place:
  > the first is the 'siphon' test – on holding the tip of the catheter above the level of insertion the fluid level or meniscus should drop to confirm negative pressure in the epidural space
  > the second is the 'aspiration test', when you aspirate through the catheter to check there is no blood or cerebrospinal fluid
  > remember that it is possible to have false negatives with these tests.
- Once you are happy with your catheter then you need to secure it in place, as the last thing you want after going to all that effort is the catheter to drop out at the end of the operation when you roll the patient!

- The final check for correct placement of the catheter is to give a test dose of local anaesthetic to ensure the catheter is not subdural. This is usually the equivalent of a spinal dose (e.g. 3 mL of 0.5% bupivacaine). If the catheter is subdural there will be evidence of a dense block usually within 5 minutes of injecting the local anaesthetic.
- Once you are happy you can then use the epidural.

Complications

It is important to be aware of these when consenting your patient as they are numerous, some common and some very rare. A recent national audit by the Royal College of Anaesthetists attempted to quantify the risk of certainly the more serious complications and it may be useful to read at least the summary so you can allow your patients to make an informed choice.[3]

- Immediate:
  > bloody tap
  > dural tap – leading to post-dural puncture headache
  > total spinal
  > high block
  > intravenous injection
  > hypotension – rarely leading to anterior spinal artery syndrome
  > nausea and vomiting
  > direct nerve trauma.
- Delayed:
  > urinary retention
  > infection or abscess
  > haematoma
  > arachnoiditis.

PERIPHERAL NERVE BLOCKS

These can be divided into:
- plexus blocks
- single nerve blocks
- plane blocks.

A description of all nerve blocks is outside the scope of this book. The important thing is that you have a general overview of the procedures including the important safety aspects and then you can learn the details of each technique as you progress in your career.

How to find the nerve?

Regional anaesthesia has gone through a renaissance of late, due to the development of ultrasound technology, which allows us to visualise even very small peripheral nerves using a small mobile machine.

Previously 'blind' techniques were used to locate the nerves, initially using anatomical landmarks and the patient noting paraesthesia and then moving on to the use of nerve stimulators to produce muscle twitches when the needle was close to the nerve. Nerve stimulators are still widely used today especially by those who do not use ultrasound routinely in their practice. They are often used in combination with ultrasound to confirm nerve location.

However, using ultrasound is slowly becoming the gold standard for peripheral nerve blockade. It is a skill in itself, which is based on a sound knowledge of anatomy and applying this to the picture produced by the ultrasound machine. It is also a technique than requires manual dexterity, good needling skills and practice, practice, practice!

The perceived advantages of ultrasound over nerve stimulators are as follows.

- The ability to see the nerve and the tissues and structures surrounding it, and therefore reducing the risk of hitting the nerve or structures such as blood vessels.
- It also allows visualisation of the spread of the local anaesthetic, reducing the amount of local anaesthetic required to block the nerve, which in turn reduces the risk of toxicity.
- It may increase the success rate for the block. However, the evidence for this is still lacking, as the technique is still in its infancy and the numbers are not large enough yet. This is very user dependent and in untrained hands the risks could be higher than the traditional blind technique!

Here are a few things to remember when using either technique.

Nerve stimulator

- These deliver an intermittent current through the needle so that as the nerve is approached the motor nerve stimulation causes muscle twitches. It is important to warn the patient, as it can be uncomfortable, especially if the current is set quite high. The patient may also complain of paraesthesia if the needle touches the nerve.
- The amount of current used is important. As the nerve is approached it should take less current to provoke a response. Once a muscle response is elicited the current is turned down. Initially the current is set at 1–1.5 mA and then reduced. The lowest point at which the twitches disappear indicates how close you are to the nerve. The twitches should disappear at 0.3 mA. Any lower than that may suggest the needle is intraneural and should be withdrawn.
- Once you start injecting the local anaesthetic the twitches should disappear. If not, then the needle tip may be beyond the nerve and should be withdrawn.
- Documentation of the currents used especially the lower threshold is vital for medico-legal purposes.

Ultrasound

- Know how to work the machine! Ideally, before using ultrasound you should attend a training course to learn the basic 'knobology' so that you know the different functions and what they are used for.
- Orientate the probe to the patient and the machine. Know which side of the screen corresponds to medial and lateral on the patient.
- Maintain asepsis – the ultrasound probe needs to be sterile for the procedure. This can be achieved with a sterile sheath (usually used for catheter insertion) or a tegaderm type dressing over the probe head.

- Ensure your ergonomics are right. Being comfortable will help prevent a shaky picture!
- Always make sure that you can visualise your injection on the screen. If you can't, then *stop*, as it may be intravascular.
- Always know where the tip of your needle is. What you think is the tip might actually be the shaft if you are slightly out of the plane of the ultrasound beam. Again, this is something that comes with practice.

Both techniques
- Asepsis is required for this technique – 2% chloraprep and sterile gloves. If you're inserting a catheter then full scrub is required.
- Regional block needles are short, bevelled and quite blunt, so it can be difficult to puncture the skin. Ensure the skin is well anaesthetised if your patient is awake. They have a short length of tubing attached, which should be primed with either local anaesthetic or normal saline. They also have a wire attached to the needle, which is plugged in to the nerve stimulator.
- If your patient is awake it is important to constantly reassure him or her, as some of the sensations can be quite unpleasant. It is also important that the patient knows to tell you if he or she has any pain or paraesthesia during the procedure, as this may indicate that you are too close to a nerve.
- A second person may inject the local anaesthetic. If you are responsible for injecting the local anaesthetic it is very important that you listen to the person who is performing the block, as they will have very specific instructions about the amount of local they wish to be injected and when.
- You should never apply excessive force during an injection. Excess pressure may be indicative of intraneural injection. If the injection feels difficult then stop and let the operator know. It is often recommended to use the same size of syringe for every block so that the 'feeling' is consistent.
- Ensure regular aspiration during injection.
- If the patient is only having a regional anaesthetic then it is important that the block is checked prior to commencing the procedure. This requires an accurate knowledge of dermotomes and myotomes. The block can be checked with either a blunt needle or ethyl chloride.

ASLEEP OR AWAKE?
This is an ongoing debate among regional anaesthetists, with some having very strong views one way or the other. Some of the points to consider are outlined here.
- Patients who are anaesthetised or heavily sedated will be unable to report paraesthesia during the block, which may indicate neuronal damage. There is no evidence currently to suggest that the incidence of neurological damage is higher in this group.
- As described earlier, verbal contact can help in the early recognition of complications, which may hasten their management.
- Most paediatric regional anaesthesia is performed asleep.
- Documentation of the presence or, more importantly absence, of paraesthesia or pain during the procedure may be useful in eliciting a cause of neurological damage further down the line.

- A very anxious or agitated patient may not tolerate the procedure while awake and actually risk more damage if he or she moves during the procedure.

See Chapter 13 for the maximum doses and duration of action of the different local anaesthetics.

Key points
- Regional techniques can provide complete anaesthesia and allow the patient to be awake during surgery, or they can provide analgesia as part of a general anaesthetic.
- Some patients and many types of surgery are unsuitable for regional anaesthesia.
- It is important that you know the safe maximum dose for local anaesthetics and that you stay below it.
- You must be able to manage local anaesthetic toxicity.
- You must be able to manage the complications of neuro-axial anaesthesia.
- You must know the anatomy of any area that you place a needle.

REFERENCES

1. Royal College of Anaesthetists. *Information for Patients*. Available at: www.rcoa.ac.uk/clinical-standards-and-quality/patient-information-leaflets (accessed 18th April 2012)
2. Cave G, Harrop-Griffiths W, Harvey M, *et al*. Management of severe local anaesthetic activity. London: Association of Anaesthetists of Great Britain and Ireland; 2010. Available at: www.aagbi.org/sites/default/files/la_toxicity_2010_0.pdf (accessed 18th April 2012)
3. Cook T. *NAP 3: major complications of central neuroaxial block in the United Kingdom*. London: Royal College of Anaesthetists; 2009.

CHAPTER 28

Stridor

VANDANA GIROTRA AND GERAINT BRIGGS

- Stridor is a loud, harsh, high-pitched respiratory sound caused by turbulent flow of air.
- It may start as low-pitched 'croaking', progressing to high-pitched 'crowing' on more vigorous respiration.
- It is caused by turbulent flow at a narrowing of a large airway.

MECHANISM

When a gas moves forward, the lateral pressure within the gas drops (the Venturi principle). In the airway, when this pressure falls, a narrowed or flexible airway (particularly so in children) collapses, obstructing airflow and generating the characteristic noise of stridor. There are three types of stridor.

1. *Inspiratory* (*extrathoracic*) stridor:
   › negative intrathoracic pressure on inspiration draws air through the narrowing, causing collapse and leading to stridor
   › expiration (positive pressure) 'pushes' the obstruction apart, reducing turbulence
   › usually caused by obstruction in upper trachea, larynx, pharynx or nose.
2. *Expiratory* (*intrathoracic*) stridor:
   › expiration 'pushes' the narrowing closer together, leading to stridor
   › negative intrathoracic pressure on inspiration 'pulls' the narrowing apart, reducing turbulent flow
   › caused by obstruction in lower trachea or bronchi.
3. *Biphasic* stridor:
   › turbulent gas flow with stridor during inspiration and expiration
   › it suggests subglottic or glottic obstruction.

An increase in the respiratory effort (e.g. increasing distress) may cause greater changes in intrathoracic pressure and airway flow rates. This exacerbates stridor and may even lead to complete airway obstruction.

CAUSES OF STRIDOR

It is important to diagnose the cause of the stridor in order to assess the risk that it poses to the patient's airway and to provide the appropriate therapy. There are many different causes of stridor that can be classified according to the patient's age and the speed of onset.

Acute stridor in children:
- congenital abnormalities
- croup or laryngotracheobronchitis
- inhaled foreign body
- epiglottitis
- anaphylaxis
- abscesses.

Chronic stridor in children:
- laryngomalacia
- subglottic stenosis
- tracheomalacia
- choanal atresia.

Acute stridor in adults:
- airway trauma
- anaphylaxis
- acute laryngitis
- aspiration of foreign body
- laryngospasm
- burns, hypocalcaemia, haematoma or oedema following neck surgery.

Chronic stridor in adults:
- Laryngeal tumour:
  › papillomatosis
  › squamous cell carcinoma.
- Laryngeal inflammation:
  › diphtheria
  › tuberculosis
  › syphilis
  › sarcoidosis.
- Tumours causing compression:
  › mediastinal tumour
  › retrosternal thyroid.
- Iatrogenic causes:
  › bronchoscopy
  › tracheal stenosis following prolonged intubation or after tracheostomy
  › neck surgery.

ASSESSMENT
History
- Onset, duration, progression and severity of symptoms
- Past medical history and details of any trauma or surgery
- Other symptoms (cough, drooling, choking, cyanosis, sleep)
- Fatigue with a decrease in stridor may signify impending respiratory arrest

Examination
- If the patient is distressed, defer further examination until equipment and facilities are available for emergency airway management.
- If acute epiglottitis is suspected, minimal examination should take place

Observe
- Fever and signs of toxicity suggesting bacterial infection
- Drooling from the mouth
- Character of cry, cough and voice
- Any positional preference that alleviates stridor

Palpate (very carefully)
- Crepitations or masses in the neck, face or chest
- Deviation of the trachea

Auscultate
- Nose, oropharynx, neck and chest (this can help locate the source of the stridor)

INVESTIGATIONS
- Mild stridor may require no investigation when self-limiting upper respiratory infections are the cause.
- Further investigations are dictated by the clinical situation, the degree of distress and the severity of the stridor.
- Pulse oximetry.
- Arterial blood gases.
- Imaging:
  - › anteroposterior and lateral X-rays of the neck and chest (particularly useful for epiglottitis)
  - › contrast studies if compression, tracheoesophageal fistula or gastro-oesophageal reflux are suspected
  - › computed tomography scanning identifies airway compression and deviation, aberrant vessels and mediastinal masses
  - › magnetic resonance imaging scanning (particularly for upper airway and vascular abnormalities)
  - › bronchoscopy.

MANAGEMENT

Call for help!

- These are complicated patients with a threatened airway and whatever your grade, you need many pairs of hands.
- You need senior anaesthetic, ENT (ear, nose and throat) and paediatric doctors.
- Never leave the patient alone.
- Interventions should be minimised if causing increasing patient distress.
- Monitoring – ideally heart rate, SpO_2, respiratory rate, blood pressure and conscious state.
- Intravenous access – ideally, prior to airway management, but may not be possible.

Medical therapy

If airway control can be delayed for a period, a number of other potential options can be considered. These include:

- oxygen by face mask, head-up position (45–90 degrees)
- nebulised epinephrine (5 mg or 5 mL 1:1000 epinephrine every 1–2 hours) in cases where airway oedema may be the cause of the stridor
- dexamethasone 4–8 mg (thrice daily) intravenously, reduces airway oedema. This takes several hours to take effect
- inhaled heliox (70% helium, 30% oxygen). Helium, being a less dense gas than nitrogen, reduces turbulent flow through narrowing in large airways. Its use may be limited by hypoxia because it only contains 30% oxygen.

Airway management

Is tracheal intubation or tracheostomy immediately necessary? This will depend on the severity of the symptoms. Severe symptoms are:

- hypoxia
- restlessness
- confusion and agitation
- ineffective respiration.

Are there signs of impending respiratory arrest?

- decreased conscious level
- reduced respiratory rate
- silent chest despite vigorous effort
- bradycardia.

If airway control cannot be delayed?

- Airway management must be led by an experienced anaesthetist with experienced help.
- The difficult airway equipment and trolley must be available.
- The ear, nose and throat surgeon should be scrubbed in case of the need for an emergency tracheostomy.
- Perform an inhalation induction using sevoflurane in 100% oxygen, carried

out in whichever position the patient is least distressed. Maintain spontaneous respiration. Disturbance of the patient *must* be minimal.

- Deep sevoflurane anaesthesia is necessary before attempting tracheal intubation.
- An endotracheal tube significantly smaller than predicted may be necessary.
- Other options would include use of halothane and awake tracheostomy.

Post-intubation care
- Transfer to critical care unit
- Adequate sedation and ventilation
- Appropriate treatment of the underlying cause (e.g. antibiotics, release of haematoma)

Key points
- Stridor can be heard at any part of the respiratory cycle.
- When it is heard it can help you diagnose the source and will aid in your medical management.
- The anaesthesia and intubation of these patients is an anaesthetic emergency and you should only attempt with help from the intensive care unit and the ear, nose and throat surgeons.

CHAPTER 29

Anaphylaxis

VANDANA GIROTRA AND GERAINT BRIGGS

Anaphylaxis is defined as a severe, life-threatening, generalised or systemic hyper-sensitivity reaction.

CLASSIFICATION

Technically, there is allergic and non-allergic anaphylaxis, but the clinical features of each may be identical. However, the treatment is the same and early identification of the mechanism will not change your practice.

- *Allergic* anaphylaxis:
  - › immunologically mediated via IgE, IgG or complement reaction.
- *Non-allergic* anaphylaxis:
  - › non-IgE mediated anaphylactic reaction. Also called an anaphylactoid reaction.

INCIDENCE DURING ANAESTHESIA

- 500 incidents in the UK per year
- 10% mortality
- Anaphylactic reactions are more common when drugs given intravenously

ANAESTHESIA-RELATED ANAPHYLAXIS

Any drug has the potential to cause an anaphylactic reaction. The commonest causes in anaesthesia are as follows.

1. Neuromuscular blocking drugs (60%):
   - › sensitisation is due to quaternary amine groups in toothpaste, detergent, shampoo, cough medicine
   - › the commonest to cause reactions is suxamethonium.
2. Latex (20%):
   - › this is most commonly found in gloves, but also in equipment such as non-invasive blood pressure cuffs
   - › the patient may report reactions prior to admission to hospital (e.g. condoms).
3. Antibiotics (15%):
   - › those with β-lactam ring account for 70%

> there is cross-sensitivity between penicillins and first-generation cephalosporins and carbapenems.
4. Colloids (4%):
    > anaphylaxis is mainly caused by gelatins, but also the starches.
5. Others:
    > non-steroidal anti-inflammatory drugs
    > chlorhexidine
    > local anaesthetics (rare)
    > opioids
    > intravenous anaesthetic agents (rare).

CLINICAL FEATURES

The clinical presentation can be very varied. No sign is pathognomonic and signs can present at different times during the anaphylaxis. The different presenting signs and their incidence are shown in Table 29.1.

TABLE 29.1 Incidence of the clinical signs of anaphylaxis

Clinical sign	Incidence (%)
Hypotension	20
Cardiovascular collapse	50
Cardiac arrest	5
Bronchospasm	40
Urticarial rash	70
Angio-oedema	12

Life-threatening problems
- *Airway*: swelling, hoarseness, stridor
- *Breathing*: wheeze, fatigue, cyanosis, SpO_2 <92%, confusion
- *Circulation*: pale, clammy, low blood pressure, faintness, drowsy or coma, cardiac arrest

MANAGEMENT[1]

Immediate management
- Remove trigger agents
- Call for help (note the time)
- Use an ABCDE (Airway, Breathing, Circulation, Disability, Exposure) approach
- Maintain and secure the airway – administer 100% oxygen
- Ventilate adequately avoiding high inspiratory airway pressures – bronchospasm requires a low respiratory rate
- Gain good intravenous access – elevate the patient's legs
- Administer adrenaline 0.5 mL of 1:10 000 solution (50 mcg increments) intravenously or 0.5 mL of 1:1000 adrenaline intramuscularly
- Administer fluids (0.9% saline or Hartmann's) 500–1000 mL

Secondary management

- Chlorpheniramine 10–20 mg intravenously or intramuscularly
- Hydrocortisone 200 mg intravenously or intramuscularly
- Adrenaline or noradrenaline infusions for persistent hypotension
- Salbutamol, aminophylline or magnesium sulphate infusions for persistent bronchospasm
- Arrange transfer to critical care

PAEDIATRIC ANAPHYLAXIS DRUG DOSES

Adrenaline

- Intramuscular:
  - › up to 6 years: 150 mcg intramuscularly (0.15 mL of 1:1000 solution)
  - › 6–12 years: 300 mcg intramuscularly (0.3 mL of 1:1000 solution)
  - › More than 12 years: 500 mcg intramuscularly (0.5 mL of 1: 1000 solution).
- Intravenous:
  - › 1 mL of 1:10 000 adrenaline for each 10 kg of body weight (0.1 mL/kg of 1:10 000 adrenaline solution = 10 mcg/kg).

Hydrocortisone

- Less than 6 months: 25 mg intramuscularly or intravenously slowly
- 6 months – 6 years: 50 mg intramuscularly or intravenously slowly
- 6–12 years: 100 mg intramuscularly or intravenously slowly
- More than 12 years: 200 mg intramuscularly or intravenously slowly

Chlorpheniramine

- Less than 6 months: 250 mcg/kg intramuscularly or intravenously slowly
- 6 months – 6 years: 2.5 mg intramuscularly or intravenously slowly
- 6–12 years: 5 mg intramuscularly or intravenously slowly
- More than 12 years: 10 mg intramuscularly or intravenously slowly

FOLLOW-UP CARE

Mast cell tryptase tests

- Take a clotted blood sample and store it in ice.
- Take the initial sample as soon as feasible. *Do not* delay resuscitation to take it.
- Second sample at 1–2 hours after the start of symptoms.
- Third sample at 24 hours or later (even in follow-up allergy clinic).
- Ensure samples are labelled with the date and time.
- Liaise with the hospital laboratory so that they are expecting the samples.

It is vital that the patient is followed up in order to ascertain the exact nature of the reaction and the causative agent. This must take place before any further anaesthesia. The most senior anaesthetist present should take responsibility for:
- reporting the reaction to the Committee on the Safety of Medicines
- documenting the reaction and liaising with the general practitioner
- arranging skin prick or intradermal allergy testing and specific IgE antibody blood testing at a specialised anaesthetic allergy clinic.

The specialist centre will require the following information in your referral:

- a legible photocopy of the anaesthetic record
- a legible photocopy of the recovery room chart
- legible photocopies of the drug charts
- a description of the reaction and time of onset in relation to induction
- details of the blood tests sent and their timing in relation to the reaction
- contact details of the surgeon and the general practitioner.

Key points

- There may be no difference in the presentation of allergic and non-allergic anaphylaxis and the treatment should be the same.
- This is a life-threatening emergency and an ABCDE approach should be used.
- Try and identify and removes potential causative agents.
- Ensure that the necessary investigations are performed and that the patient is referred to an allergy clinic for follow-up.

REFERENCE

1. Association of Anaesthetists of Great Britain and Ireland (2009). *Suspected Anaphylactic Reactions Associated with Anaesthesia.* Anaesthesia, 64, 199–211. Also available at www.aagbi. org. UK Resuscitation Council Guidelines. www.resus.org.uk.

FURTHER READING

- Mertes PM, Laxenaire MC, Alla F; Groupe d'Etudes des Réactions Anaphylactoïdes Peranesthésiques. Clinical features of allergic anaphylaxis and non-allergic anaphylaxis occurring during anaesthesia in France between 1st Jan 1999 and 31st Dec 2000. *Anesthesiology.* 2003; **99**(3): 536–45.

CHAPTER 30

Major haemorrhage

NATALIE COOPER AND STEVEN BENINGTON

Major haemorrhage has various definitions relating to transfusion requirements, including:

- replacement of the circulating volume in a 24-hour period
- blood transfusion exceeding six units of packed red cells
- acute administration of over 1.5 times the patient's blood volume.

Defining major haemorrhage is far less important than recognising its presence and reacting quickly and efficiently. It may be obvious (e.g. blood filling up the suction bottle in theatre during a vascular case) or occult requiring a high index of suspicion (e.g. a trauma patient in the emergency department developing signs of shock).

Major haemorrhage is a critical incident requiring urgent intervention.

One anaesthetist alone, however experienced, cannot manage it and help should be obtained at the earliest opportunity.

This chapter makes frequent reference to the Association of Anaesthetists of Great Britain and Ireland guidelines on major haemorrhage.[1] Each trust will have its own major haemorrhage protocol, detailing how to access the appropriate help and prompt availability of blood products in an emergency situation, and it is important to be familiar with this.

RECOGNITION AND ASSESSMENT

Prompt recognition of haemorrhage is essential; successful haemostasis depends on stopping the source of blood loss while maintaining blood coagulation as near normal as possible. If blood loss continues, the patient loses clotting factors and becomes hypothermic, while organs become underperfused, oxygen delivery falls and shock supervenes with a metabolic acidosis.

The extent of haemorrhage may be obvious in theatre where blood loss can be monitored (but beware underestimating losses contained in blood-soaked swabs), but it can be more difficult in other environments and a high index of suspicion is important. Even apparently minor abdominal trauma can cause catastrophic bleeding from the liver or spleen, and the thoracic cavity, pelvis and long bones should always be assessed clinically and radiologically.

Table 30.1 is adapted from the Advanced Trauma Life Support program for Doctors manual[2] and gives a framework for the assessment of a patient's haemorrhage; it serves as a useful reminder of the features of hypovolaemic shock. Any patient in class 3 and above will almost certainly need blood transfusion, but a patient with class 1 shock and ongoing bleeding also needs prompt attention to prevent further haemorrhage.

TABLE 30.1 Classification of haemorrhagic shock (adapted from American College of Surgeons Committee on Trauma[2])

	Class 1	Class 2	Class 3	Class 4
Blood loss (%)	<15	15–30	30–40	>40
Heart rate (bpm)	Normal	>100	>120	>140
Pulse pressure	Normal	Decreased	Decreased	Decreased
Systolic blood pressure	Normal	Decreased	Decreased	Decreased (preterminal)
Respiratory rate (breaths per minute)	14–20	20–30	30–40	>35
Urine output	Normal	20–30 mL/hour	5–15 mL/hour	Negligible
Conscious level	Slightly anxious	Mildly anxious	Anxious, confused	Confused, lethargic

IMMEDIATE MANAGEMENT

Once major haemorrhage is recognised the local major haemorrhage protocol should be activated. This will involve a coordinated response from different members of the hospital team including:

- blood bank
- haematologist
- porter
- senior anaesthetist or clinician on duty, depending on the location
- theatre staff or nursing staff, depending on location.

Once alerted, blood bank can prepare suitable blood products depending on the urgency of the situation.

- Blood products should be ordered as early as possible, since fresh frozen plasma (FFP) and cryoprecipitate take 30 minutes to defrost.
- Group-specific blood can usually be issued within 15 minutes of receiving a sample, and this should be requested if possible to preserve the scarce O-negative supply.
- Fully cross-matched blood takes up to 45 minutes.
- If blood is required immediately then group O-negative should be requested. A small supply of O-negative packed red cells is usually maintained in emergency care areas for this use, including emergency theatre, obstetric theatre and the emergency department.

It is increasingly recognised that replacement of clotting factors and platelets should be commenced early rather than waiting for a significant coagulopathy to develop. Therefore, most hospitals have a major haemorrhage 'shock pack' containing:

- packed red cells (4–6 units)
- FFP (4 units)
- platelets (one adult dose), which can be requested from blood bank for immediate use.

Many of the following points can be performed simultaneously by different members of the team under the direction of a team leader. One person should be dedicated to administrative duties, including ordering blood products, documentation and liaising with other specialities as required.

Haemorrhage control

- Obvious bleeding points must be controlled with direct pressure and elevation where possible.
- Surgery may be required for definitive haemorrhage control, with simultaneous resuscitation provided by the anaesthetist.
- A gastroenterologist or endoscopist may be required for major gastrointestinal haemorrhage.
- An interventional radiologist may be able to embolise the arterial supply to otherwise difficult to control sources of bleeding such as hepatic injury.

ABC assessment and oxygen

- ABC (Airway, Breathing, Circulation) assessment and oxygen should be performed according to adult life support principles, with oxygen applied at 15L/minute via a non-rebreathe mask in the emergency situation, and subsequently titrated to saturations and arterial PaO_2.

Intravenous access

- Intravenous access should be with large-bore cannula (ideally two 14–16 G cannulae peripherally).
- Flow through a large-bore peripheral cannula is far greater than through a standard central line and time should not be wasted inserting the latter to the exclusion of other activities.
- If intravenous access is difficult, intraosseous access should be attempted for initial fluid resuscitation. Intravenous access can be gained once circulating volume is restored.

Bloods

- Following cannulation, blood should be sent for:
  - cross-match
  - full blood count
  - coagulation screen
  - fibrinogen.
- Near-patient testing is invaluable if available, with arterial blood gas analysis and thromboelastography giving early and reliable information on haemoglobin and haemostatic function.

Intravenous fluid resuscitation

- While awaiting blood products it is reasonable to infuse intravenous crystalloid or colloid to maintain tissue perfusion.
- It is recognised that overenthusiastic fluid resuscitation with the aim of normotension may increase bleeding through disruption of clot that has formed at the traumatised area. For this reason, *prior* to definitive haemostasis a lower blood pressure should be targeted.
- In practice, if the (non-anaesthetised) patient is talking and has a peripheral pulse this is an adequate end point ('hypotensive resuscitation').
- The presence of a palpable radial pulse implies a systolic blood pressure of at least 80 mmHg.
- Once definitive haemostasis has been secured, normotension should be the aim to improve tissue perfusion and reverse the effects of hypovolaemic shock.
- In patients with a head injury, hypotensive resuscitation should not be practised, since normotension is required to optimise cerebral perfusion and avoid worsening the brain injury.

Active warming

- Hypothermia develops rapidly in haemorrhaging patients and can contribute to coagulopathy and the 'lethal triad'. Patients should be warmed with forced air warmers and all fluids, particularly blood, should be warmed via a suitable device.
- Attention should be given to other sources of heat loss, including the ambient temperature.

Imaging

- If the source of the haemorrhage is unclear (e.g. following polytrauma or in the case of a suspected but unconfirmed ruptured abdominal aortic aneurysm), further imaging is desirable. This may be in the form of plain radiography, ultrasound at the bedside or involve transfer for a computed tomography scan.
- The decision to take such patients to the radiology department should not be taken lightly, and a haemodynamically unstable patient may be better served by immediate laparotomy if an abdominal source of blood loss is suspected.
- Occasionally transfer to the radiology department may be therapeutic as well as diagnostic (if embolisation is planned).
- Such decisions should be taken by senior surgical and anaesthetic personnel.

Alert theatre and cell salvage

- If the patient is not already in theatre, then the department should be informed as soon as possible regarding any potential surgical cases so that they can prepare for the patient's arrival.
- Staff competent in the use of intra-operative cell salvage should also be contacted urgently.
- Cell salvage can reduce allogenic blood requirements, but does not prevent coagulopathy because the blood is washed and filtered prior to reinfusion, which removes clotting factors.

MANAGEMENT OF COAGULOPATHY

Coagulopathy is common in major haemorrhage and is usually caused by coagulation factor dilution. In some patients it may also be due to drugs (e.g. anticoagulants, antiplatelet agents) or a consumptive coagulopathy (i.e. disseminated intravascular coagulation). Coagulopathy should be anticipated in any patient with massive haemorrhage undergoing transfusion, and should be treated proactively rather than reactively.

For blood to form a clot it needs coagulation factors, fibrinogen and platelets. If any of these are deficient then clotting will be deranged. Therefore, all these factors need replacing during major haemorrhage.

- FFP is rich in clotting factors and the early use of 15 mL/kg is recommended and more than 30 mL/kg is advocated if haemostatic failure is evident.
- Platelets are often held in a central site, which can be far from the hospital, and should be requested early.
- Fibrinogen should also be replaced with either cryoprecipitate or fibrinogen concentrate (30–60 mg/kg) depending on local protocols.
- Some trusts will issue 'shock packs' as described earlier, which are designed to provide the necessary coagulation products with each order of packed red cells.

Regular coagulation testing should be performed to assess the response to treatment. Laboratory testing takes time and therefore near-patient testing, such as thromboelastography is useful in providing early information. Liaison with a senior haematologist is also essential. Suggested parameters for adequate haemostasis include:

- prothrombin time and activated partial thromboplastin time ratio <1.5 times normal
- platelet count >75 × 10^3/mm^3
- fibrinogen >1.5 g/L.

Drugs that should be considered include the following.

- *Ionised calcium* (in the form of calcium chloride or calcium gluconate): hypocalcaemia is common in massive transfusions and ionised calcium is required for haemostasis; therefore, it is advisable to monitor and correct it. Most blood gas analysers provide a value for ionised calcium.
- *Tranexamic acid*: this is an antifibrinolytic drug that can be given as a loading dose of 1 g over 10 minutes followed by 1 g over 8 hours. It reduces the risk of death when given early in bleeding trauma patients,[3] and may well benefit other bleeding patient groups.
- *Recombinant factor VIIa*: this extremely expensive drug can be anecdotally effective in treating massive haemorrhage, but the evidence base for its use in major trauma is limited at present, and it is unlicensed for this indication. The Association of Anaesthetists of Great Britain and Ireland guidelines recommend that local protocols should be followed and it should be given with tranexamic acid.[1] The decision to use it will normally be made in conjunction with a senior haematologist.

FURTHER MANAGEMENT

Stabilisation

- Once haemorrhage is controlled, the patient's blood pressure should be maintained at normal levels and his or her acid base status should be assessed and addressed.
- Hypothermia should be managed with continued active warming.
- Arrangements should be made for the patient to be cared for in a critical care area post-operatively.
- Blood tests including full blood count, urea and electrolytes, coagulation screen, fibrinogen and blood gases should be monitored regularly.

Thromboprophylaxis

- Following massive haemorrhage patients can become prothrombotic and venous thromboprophylaxis should be instituted when safe. This includes mechanical methods such as compression stockings and intermittent calf compression devices.
- The use of low-molecular-weight heparin should be discussed with a surgeon and haematologist in order that the risks of bleeding versus thrombosis are balanced.

Key points

- Major haemorrhage is a critical incident requiring a multidisciplinary team approach.
- The key to a successful outcome is to involve the relevant people early and to have good communication throughout.
- Source control is essential and may require a surgeon, gastroenterologist or interventional radiologist.
- Coagulopathy should be anticipated and treated early and aggressively, with regular blood tests and near-patient testing used as a guide.
- Each hospital should have a major haemorrhage protocol and this should be familiar to all healthcare professionals involved in the care of a bleeding patient.

REFERENCES

1. Thomas D, Wee M, Clyburn P, *et al.* Association of Anaesthetists of Great Britain and Ireland. Blood transfusion and the anaesthetist: management of massive haemorrhage. *Anaesthesia.* 2010; **65**(11): 1153–61.
2. American College of Surgeons Committee on Trauma. *Advanced Trauma Life Support Program for Doctors.* Chicago. American College of Surgeons. 2004; Chapter 3 Shock p. 69–102.
3. Shakur H, Roberts I, Bautista R, *et al.* CRASH-2 Trial Collaborators. Effects of tranexamic acid on death, vascular occlusive events, and blood transfusion in trauma patients with significant haemorrhage (CRASH-2): a randomised, placebo-controlled trial. *Lancet.* 2010; **376**(9734): 23–32.

CHAPTER 31

Rapid sequence induction at a remote site

NITIN ARORA

Most rapid sequence inductions by anaesthetic trainees will be performed in the theatre complex. However, there may be occasions when you have to perform a rapid sequence induction at a site distant from theatres. A remote site is defined as a location outside the theatre complex where assistance from another anaesthetist is not immediately available. These places may include:

- the emergency department
- the coronary care unit
- the radiology department
- medical or surgical wards
- intensive care.

Of these locations, intensive care may appear to be safe but it may not have enough staff members who are trained in anaesthetic procedures. There are many problems associated with anaesthesia at a remote site. These may include:

- non-availability of trained help
- lack of immediate supervision
- poor lighting
- limited availability of drugs, ventilator and airway equipment
- absence of specialised equipment (e.g. difficult intubation trolley).

These patients may be deteriorating rapidly and need airway control for a variety of reasons. In many cases, the safest course of action may be to transfer the patient to the theatre suite. However, sometimes, there may not be enough time to transfer the patient and you may be forced to start the rapid sequence induction in an unfamiliar location.

The first consideration in this situation must be patient safety.

SUPERVISION

You must ensure you have adequate supervision. This may be direct, local or distant supervision depending on the clinical situation and your experience and competence. *If in doubt, call your senior*. All anaesthetics at a remote site must have a named consultant.

HELP

A safe anaesthetic must not be conducted in the absence of trained assistance. This should normally be an operating department practitioner (ODP) from theatres. ODPs can be worth their weight in gold. If a good ODP suggests something, *listen!*

You will need an ODP or anaesthetic nurse to help you set up equipment and monitoring and to provide cricoid pressure.

DRUGS

You must ensure you have the required medication available before you start. This will include the following.

- *Drugs for induction*: will normally be an induction agent (e.g. thiopentone sodium) and a muscle relaxant (typically, suxamethonium).
- *Drugs to keep the patient asleep*: an opioid (usually morphine or alfentanil), a hypnotic (e.g. propofol or midazolam) and a muscle relaxant (e.g. atracurium).
- *Emergency drugs*: such as vasopressors (e.g. metaraminol), anticholinergics (e.g. atropine or glycopyrronium) and adrenaline.

MONITORING AND EQUIPMENT

The Association of Anaesthetists of Great Britain and Ireland sets out minimum monitoring standards for anaesthesia in the UK and these must be followed. Electrocardiograph, pulse oximetry and blood pressure monitoring should be available almost everywhere. Capnography may be more difficult, but in view of the new resuscitation guidelines, all locations should have access to capnography soon.

The need for suction and a tilting trolley or bed must not be forgotten.

Also, make sure you have assessed the patient's airway and readied the airway equipment, which should include, at the very minimum, a couple of working laryngoscopes with blades, a selection of endotracheal tubes, a bougie and a laryngeal mask for rescue.

If the airway looks tricky, ask for help and get the difficult airway trolley (or even better, relocate to theatres).

Don't forget that you will have to breathe for the patient. This will need a portable ventilator or manual ventilation with a self-inflating bag or a Mapleson C circuit.

Once you have managed to complete the induction of anaesthesia, take a deep breath and carry on with stabilising the patient. An ABCDE (Airway, Breathing, Circulation, Disability, Exposure) approach often works best!

The patient will then need to be transferred to a safer location.

Key points

- Whenever you are away from the anaesthetic room there will be less help and less equipment.
- The key is preparation, planning and asking for help early.
- You must decide if it is safer and more practical to take the patient to the anaesthetic room.
- Ensure that you still follow the Association of Anaesthetists of Great Britain and Ireland guidelines for monitoring.

FURTHER READING

- *The Royal College of Anaesthetists Guidelines on Anaesthetic Services at a Remote Site.* London: Royal College of Anaesthetists 2011. Available at: www.rcoa.ac.uk/document-store/anaesthetic-services-remote-sites (accessed 24 April 2013).
- Cook TM, Woodall N, Frerk C; Fourth National Audit Project. Major complications of airway management in the UK: results of the Fourth National Audit Project of the Royal College of Anaesthetists and the Difficult Airway Society. Part 1: anaesthesia. *Br J Anaesth.* 2011; **106**(5): 617–31.
- Cook TM, Woodall N, Harper J, *et al.* Fourth National Audit Project. Major complications of airway management in the UK: results of the Fourth National Audit Project of the Royal College of Anaesthetists and the Difficult Airway Society. Part 2: intensive care and emergency departments. *Br J Anaesth.* 2011; **106**(5): 632–42.

CHAPTER 32

Asthma and anaesthesia

TINA DUFF

Asthma is a disease characterised by reversible airflow obstruction. Narrowing of the airways is provoked by inflammation of hypertrophied bronchial smooth muscle, bronchial mucosal oedema and extensive eosinophil infiltration, all of which contribute to bronchoconstriction. Asthma is also associated with hypersecretion from the mucous-producing cells lining the airways, which results in excessive thick and tenacious secretions that can lead to blocked distal airways and gas trapping. These pathological mechanisms lead to:

- high airways resistance
- hypoxaemia
- an increase in the work of breathing
- this can eventually lead to exhaustion and the need for intubation and ventilation.

ASSESSING A PATIENT WITH ASTHMA

As an anaesthetist you are going to encounter hundreds of patients with asthma. It is important that you carefully assess each of these patients to ascertain their risks of undergoing anaesthesia and establish the best plan for delivering your anaesthetic.

Remember that the patient is usually the best judge of his or her asthma and how well it is currently controlled. Some patients will be able to tell you what their best peak flow measurement is and how they are currently performing. Some patients may even have a peak flow diary. Often those patients who keep a peak flow diary have difficult to control asthma, so perhaps think of this as a red flag. It is vital that you use your preoperative visit to establish how severe a patient's asthma has been in the past and what triggers can induce a deterioration in the control of his or her asthma. Questions you need to ask are:

- What medications are you currently taking for asthma?
- How frequently do you require your preventative inhaler?
- Do you have home nebulisers?
- How frequently do you take oral steroids?
- Have you ever been admitted to hospital with your asthma?
- If you were admitted to hospital did you require admission to the high dependency unit (HDU) or the intensive care unit (ICU)?

- Have you been intubated and ventilated because of your asthma in the past?
- What triggers your asthma attacks?
- Can you do strenuous activities/What is your exercise tolerance?
- Do you have any allergies?
- Do non-steroidal anti-inflammatory drugs (aspirin, ibuprofen) make your asthma worse?
- Has your asthma deteriorated over the last few weeks or months?
- Have you had any recent coryzal (runny nose, sore throat) symptoms?
- Do you have a nocturnal cough? (This can be a good indication of poorly controlled asthma).

Single peak flow measurements are not as informative as serial measurements; however, single measurements can be compared with a patient's normal reading or predicted values based on height, weight and sex to give an impression of the respiratory function of a patient. Examination is frequently normal and a chest X-ray (CXR) is not necessary. Blood gas analysis is only useful in assessing patients with severe asthma prior to major surgery.

Having seen a patient preoperatively you should then be able to establish whether you think he or she is high or low risk.

WHICH ANAESTHETIC?

There is never a single right answer to the question, 'what anaesthetic should this patient receive?' It is good practice to have several different plans in place for each patient, as things do not always go as anticipated. In severe asthmatics undergoing major abdominal or thoracic surgery a bed on the HDU or the ICU should be available for post-operative monitoring.

The elective asthmatic patient

Asthma is very commonly exacerbated by viral infections; therefore, if there is any evidence of an upper respiratory tract infection then postponing surgery should be considered.

Another reason to postpone elective surgery is poorly controlled asthma; this may be manifest by highly variable peak flow readings, nocturnal coughing and high use of preventative medications. It is clearly important in this situation to either (1) write to the general practitioner or (2) arrange a clinic appointment with a respiratory physician to enable optimisation of medical therapy.

You will need to discuss these two situations with the anaesthetic consultant in charge, as cancelling patients is a senior decision.

The emergency asthmatic patient

An emergency operation in a poorly controlled or severe asthmatic can be very challenging. Therefore, it is essential to ask for help and to discuss the alternative anaesthetic techniques that could be utilised in such cases.

Regional anaesthesia is often a suitable technique in asthmatic patients. However, this relies on the operative site being amenable to regional anaesthesia and the consent of the patient.

There will be many cases where a general anaesthetic is necessary. Therefore, it is essential to undertake optimisation of the patient as quickly as possible and to use the safest possible anaesthetic technique. If possible, tracheal intubation can be avoided by using a laryngeal mask. If tracheal intubation is essential then we need to minimise the risks of bronchospasm.

Optimise the patient's asthma

There is usually only a limited amount of time for optimisation in an emergency but there is time for the administration of nebulised β_2-adrenoreceptor agonists and nebulised anticholinergic medications. In severe cases you can also consider oral or intravenous steroids. Physiotherapy can be useful.

In elective cases patients should bring their preventative inhalers to the anaesthetic room, where many anaesthetists will ask them to have their normal inhaled dose.

Limiting bronchospasm

As already discussed, avoiding tracheal intubation is the best way of avoiding bronchospasm; however, this is often unavoidable. It is important to recognise that many of the drugs that we use in our everyday anaesthetic practice may cause or exacerbate bronchospasm by the release of histamine:

- morphine
- atracurium
- mivacurium
- thiopentone.

Drugs that are considered safe include:

- propofol
- ketamine
- etomidate
- midazolam
- pethidine
- fentanyl
- alfentanil
- vecuronium
- rocuronium
- suxamethonium
- volatile agents (sevoflurane should be used for a gas induction).

Intubation may be the most potent stimulus to bronchospasm; therefore, it is vitally important that intubation is carried out under adequate anaesthesia usually with opioid cover. Other techniques used to reduce bronchospasm at intubation include the use of 1–2 mg/kg of lidocaine intravenously or application of lidocaine to the cords using an atomiser spray. Avoid dehydration.

Extubation

It is not uncommon to cause bronchospasm at extubation. Therefore, it is essential to plan as carefully for extubation as intubation. Ensure adequate analgesia has been administered and all paralytic agents are completely reversed. There are then two different approaches to extubation: (1) deep and (2) awake extubation.

- In an elective case where there is no risk of aspiration you can plan to undertake a deep extubation, otherwise we should be aiming to extubate when the patient is awake (*see* Chapter 10 Airway management).
- Awake extubation can be difficult as disturbing the patient during the light planes of anaesthesia can precipitate the development of laryngospasm and bronchospasm.
- Therefore, it is good practice to suction the pharynx and larynx under deep anaesthesia and then not to disturb the patient until he or she is awake and extubatable.
- All the equipment for reintubation should be immediately available.

It is now possible to administer metered dose inhalers via the anaesthetic circuit without interruption. The administration of six to ten puffs of salbutamol can be considered prior to extubation.

ACUTE BRONCHOSPASM OR AN EXACERBATION OF ASTHMA

Acute bronchospasm may occur at any time. It is clearly different identifying bronchospasm during anaesthesia than it is in an awake patient.

Bronchospasm during surgery

Bronchospasm can be detected clinically by auscultation of the chest. It may be possible to hear a prolonged expiratory wheeze, but in severe cases there may be a 'silent chest' as a result of minimal air movement. Disconnecting the breathing circuit may allow you to hear an expiratory wheeze through the endotracheal tube.

Monitoring will also help you identify possible bronchospasm. Airway pressure will rise and tidal volumes will reduce during intermittent positive pressure ventilation. The capnograph trace will show a rising end-tidal carbon dioxide measurement as well as a prolonged and upsloping expiratory trace.

In a ventilated patient, airway obstruction due to bronchospasm may be difficult to diagnose. Alternative reasons for airflow obstruction include:

- breathing circuit obstruction
- anaphylaxis
- pneumothorax
- foreign body (including aspiration)
- irritation of the carina or endobronchial intubation.

The quickest way to assess for bronchospasm is to disconnect the breathing circuit and the filter and to manually ventilate using a self-inflating bag or a Mapleson C circuit attached at the alternative oxygen source.

- If the airway pressures remain high, ensure the endotracheal tube is not blocked by passing a suction catheter or bougie and measuring the distance until resistance.
- If airway pressures are still high, bronchospasm is the most likely explanation.

Bronchospasm in an awake patient

An exacerbation of asthma is classified in the *British Guideline on the Management of Asthma*[1] as:

- moderate
- acute severe
- life-threatening
- near fatal.

Acute severe asthma is any one of:
- peak expiratory flow of 33%–50% best or predicted
- respiratory rate ≥25 breaths per minute
- heart rate ≥110 beats per minute
- inability to complete sentences in one breath.

In life-threatening asthma you have to have evidence of acute severe asthma and any one of:
- peak expiratory flow of <33% best or predicted
- SpO_2 <92%
- PaO_2 <8 kPa
- normal $PaCO_2$ (4.6–6.0 kPa)
- silent chest
- cyanosis
- poor respiratory effort
- arrhythmia
- exhaustion, altered conscious level.

It is imperative that you are aware of these British guidelines and the classification system used, as well as the recommended management of acute asthma.

THE MANAGEMENT OF ACUTE BRONCHOSPASM
The management of bronchospasm should be second nature to you. There are obviously variations depending on the setting of the patient.

The intubated and ventilated patient in theatre
- Get help
- Ask the surgeon to stop operating
- 100% oxygen
- Increase the inspired concentration of volatile anaesthetic, or consider its introduction if using total intravenous anaesthesia
- Check the position of the endotracheal tube, and exclude a pneumothorax – order a CXR
- Administer a β_2 agonist via a metered-dose inhaler or a nebuliser
- Hydrocortisone 200 mg (if not already on high-dose steroids)
- Consider intravenous salbutamol 250 µg as a slow bolus
- Consider 1.2–2 g of magnesium intravenously
- Ipratropium bromide nebuliser
- Ketamine 2 mg/kg intravenously can be used in severe bronchospasm
- Patients who do not respond to initial treatments may require a salbutamol infusion or an aminophylline infusion (a salbutamol infusion is first line in the *British Guidelines on the Management of Asthma*;[1] however, some patients,

particularly those on regular oral theophylline may respond well to an aminophylline infusion) – if a patient is already on oral theophylline no loading dose of aminophylline is required
- Arterial blood gases will help guide your management – an arterial line may be helpful.

In severe bronchospasm, gas trapping may cause a reduction in venous return and a reduced cardiac output. It may be necessary to regularly disconnect the patient from the breathing circuit and apply pressure to the thorax to manually expel the gas. It is often easier in severe bronchospasm to manually ventilate the patient until there is an improvement. This enables you to deliver a slow rate, with a long expiratory time to allow for prolonged expiration seen in this condition. Initially there may be a marked rise in the expired carbon dioxide levels but this is allowable as long as oxygenation is maintained (permissive hypercapnia).

It is also important to ensure that you exclude anaphylaxis as a cause of broncho-spasm, immediately stop any drug being administered that may precipitate anaphylaxis and review the drug chart for any other possible causes. (If anaphylaxis is suspected then manage appropriately as per the anaphylaxis algorithm.)

You will need to arrange for this patient to be transferred to ICU if his or her bron-chospasm has been very difficult to control or is still requiring treatment.

A patient in recovery post-operatively
Assess the severity of the patient's asthma using the criteria described earlier while instituting immediate management.
- Get appropriate help.
- Humidified 100% oxygen.
- Salbutamol via a metered-dose inhaler or nebuliser.
- Back-to-back nebulisers.
- Hydrocortisone 200 mg intravenously or prednisolone 40 mg orally (if not already on high-dose steroids).
- Examine the patient and aim to exclude a pneumothorax and the presence of an urticarial rash – order a CXR.
- Consider magnesium 1.2–2 g intravenously.
- Consider intravenous salbutamol 250 μg as a slow bolus.
- An arterial blood gas analysis will be helpful in assessing the severity of the asthma/bronchospasm.
- Consider either a salbutamol infusion or an aminophylline infusion if the bronchospasm is not controlled with the immediate measures described. Aminophylline may be more appropriate in patients who are already taking regular oral theophylline.
- If the patient continues to deteriorate then it is important to ask for a critical care review, as intubation may be necessary or close observation in a critical care area.

Refer to the *British Guidelines on the Management of Asthma*[1] for the recommended treatment of adults and children of different ages. The information in this chapter is in reference to adults only.

POST-OPERATIVE CARE OF THE ASTHMATIC PATIENT

As discussed earlier, for patients with severe asthma who are undergoing major abdominal or thoracic surgery, a post-operative bed on HDU or ICU should be secured before starting the procedure. These patients benefit from good analgesia, which will often be provided by an epidural.

It is also important to ensure that asthmatic patients who are returning to the ward do not get into avoidable difficulty. If a patient is going to be nil by mouth then regular oral medications should be changed to an intravenous form – in particular, steroid treatment. Adequate pain control must be prescribed and regional techniques are often useful in supplementing analgesia. If non-steroidal anti-inflammatory drugs or other medications exacerbate a patient's asthma, ensure this is clearly documented on the drugs chart.

Adequate hydration is also essential. Check the fluid prescription chart and if the patient's fluids are due to run out in the middle of the night, write up another bag.

Prescribe regular β_2-agonists via a metered-dose inhaler or nebuliser. If it is on the as-required part of the prescription it will not be given. The dose can be de-escalated as required.

> **Key points**
> - Asthma is a condition that you will encounter frequently.
> - You need to assess a patient with asthma and establish his or her risks for anaesthesia.
> - Always have several different plans for your anaesthetic, as you never know what may happen.
> - If at all possible try to avoid tracheal intubation by the use of regional techniques or laryngeal masks.
> - Ensure post-operative plans are in place.
> - Keep up to date with the management of acute asthma or bronchospasm, as you need to act quickly when dealing with these situations.
> - Always ask for help in emergency situations.

REFERENCE

1. The British Thoracic Society. *British Guideline on the Management of Asthma*. Guideline No. 101. Edinburgh: Scottish Intercollegiate Guidelines Network; 2011.

Management of a patient with suspected anaphylaxis during anaesthesia – safety drill

THE ASSOCIATION OF ANAESTHETISTS
of Great Britain & Ireland

Management of a Patient with Suspected Anaphylaxis During Anaesthesia
SAFETY DRILL

(Revised 2009)

Immediate management

- Use the ABC approach (Airway, Breathing, and Circulation). Team-working enables several tasks to be accomplished simultaneously.

- Remove all potential causative agents and maintain anaesthesia, if necessary, with an inhalational agent.

- **CALL FOR HELP** and note the time.

- Maintain the airway and administer oxygen 100%. Intubate the trachea if necessary and ventilate the lungs with oxygen.

- Elevate the patient's legs if there is hypotension.

- If appropriate, start cardiopulmonary resuscitation immediately according to Advanced Life Support Guidelines.

- Give adrenaline i.v.

  - Adult dose: 50 µg (0.5 ml of 1:10 000 solution).
  - Child dose: 1.0 µg.kg^{-1} (0.1 ml.kg^{-1} 1:100 000 solution).

- Several doses may be required if there is severe hypotension or bronchospasm. If several doses of adrenaline are required, consider starting an intravenous infusion of adrenaline.

- Give saline 0.9% or lactated Ringer's solution at a high rate via an intravenous cannula of an appropriate gauge (large volumes may be required).

  - Adult: 500 - 1 000 ml
  - Child: 20 ml.kg^{-1}

- Plan transfer of the patient to an appropriate Critical Care area.

CONTINUED OVERLEAF

Secondary management

· Give chlorphenamine i.v.

Adult:	10 mg
Child 6 - 12 years:	5 mg
Child 6 months - 6 years:	2.5 mg
Child <6 months:	250 µg.kg^{-1}

· Give hydrocortisone i.v.

Adult:	200 mg
Child 6 - 12 years:	100 mg
Child 6 months - 6 years:	50 mg
Child <6 months:	25 mg

· If the blood pressure does not recover despite an adrenaline infusion, consider the administration of an alternative i.v. vasopressor according to the training and experience of the anaesthetist, e.g. metaraminol.

· Treat persistent bronchospasm with an i.v. infusion of salbutamol. If a suitable breathing system connector is available, a metered-dose inhaler may be appropriate. Consider giving i.v. aminophylline or magnesium sulphate.

Investigation

· Take blood samples (5 - 10 ml clotted blood) for **mast cell tryptase** :

  ◦ Initial sample as soon as feasible after resuscitation has started – do not delay resuscitation to take the sample.

  ◦ Second sample at 1 - 2 h after the start of symptoms.

  ◦ Third sample either at 24 h or in convalescence (for example in a follow-up allergy clinic). This is a measure of baseline tryptase levels as some individuals have a higher baseline level.

· Ensure that the samples are labelled with the time and date.

· Liaise with the hospital laboratory about analysis of samples.

Later investigations to identify the causative agent

The anaesthetist who gave the anaesthetic or the supervising consultant anaesthetist is responsible for ensuring that the reaction is investigated. The patient should be referred to a specialist Allergy or Immunology Centre (see www.aagbi.org for details). The patient, surgeon and general practitioner should be informed. Reactions should be notified to the AAGBI National Anaesthetic Anaphylaxis Database (see www.aagbi.org).

This guideline is not to be construed as a standard of medical care. Standards of medical care are determined on the basis of all clinical data available for an individual case and are subject to change as knowledge advances. The ultimate judgement with regard to a particular clinical procedure or treatment plan must be made by the clinician in light of the clinical data presented and the diagnostic and treatment options available.

© The Association of Anaesthetists of Great Britain & Ireland 2009

Checklist for anaesthetic equipment 2012 – AAGBI safety guideline

Checklist for Anaesthetic Equipment 2012
AAGBI Safety Guideline

Checks at the start of every operating session
Do not use this equipment unless you have been trained

Check self-inflating bag available

Perform manufacturer's (automatic) machine check

Power supply	• Plugged in • Switched on • Back-up battery charged
Gas supplies and suction	• Gas and vacuum pipelines – 'tug test' • Cylinders filled and turned off • Flowmeters working (if applicable) • Hypoxic guard working • Oxygen flush working • Suction clean and working
Breathing system	• Whole system patent and leak free using 'two-bag' test • Vaporisers – fitted correctly, filled, leak free, plugged in (if necessary) • Soda lime - colour checked • Alternative systems (Bain, T-piece) – checked • Correct gas outlet selected
Ventilator	• Working and configured correctly
Scavenging	• Working and configured correctly
Monitors	• Working and configured correctly • Alarms limits and volumes set
Airway equipment	• Full range required, working, with spares

RECORD THIS CHECK IN THE PATIENT RECORD

Don't Forget!	• Self-inflating bag • Common gas outlet • Difficult airway equipment • Resuscitation equipment • TIVA and/or other infusion equipment

CHECKS BEFORE EACH CASE

Breathing system	Whole system patent and leak free using 'two-bag' test Vaporisers – fitted correctly, filled, leak free, plugged in (if necessary) Alternative systems (Bain, T-piece) – checked Correct gas outlet selected
Ventilator	Working and configured correctly
Airway equipment	Full range required, working, with spares
Suction	Clean and working

THE TWO-BAG TEST

A two-bag test should be performed after the breathing system, vaporisers and ventilator have been checked individually

i.   Attach the patient end of the breathing system (including angle piece and filter) to a test lung or bag.

ii. Set the fresh gas flow to 5 l.min^{-1} and ventilate manually. Check the whole breathing system is patent and the unidirectional valves are moving. Check the function of the APL valve by squeezing both bags.

iii. Turn on the ventilator to ventilate the test lung. Turn off the fresh gas flow, or reduce to a minimum. Open and close each vaporiser in turn. There should be no loss of volume in the system.

This checklist is an abbreviated version of the publication by the Association of Anaesthetists of Great Britain and Ireland 'Checking Anaesthesia Equipment 2012'. It was originally published in *Anaesthesia*.
(Endorsed by the Chief Medical Officers)

If you wish to refer to this guideline, please use the following reference: Checklist for anaesthetic equipment 2012. *Anaesthesia* 2012; **66:** pages 662–63. http://onlinelibrary.wiley.com/doi/10.1111/j.1365-2044.2012.07163.x/abstract

AAGBI safety guideline – management of severe local anaesthetic toxicity

AAGBI Safety Guideline
Management of Severe Local Anaesthetic Toxicity

1 **Recognition**	**Signs of severe toxicity:** • Sudden alteration in mental status, severe agitation or loss of consciousness, with or without tonic-clonic convulsions • Cardiovascular collapse: sinus bradycardia, conduction blocks, asystole and ventricular tachyarrhythmias may all occur • Local anaesthetic (LA) toxicity may occur some time after an initial injection
2 **Immediate management**	• Stop injecting the LA • Call for help • Maintain the airway and, if necessary, secure it with a tracheal tube • Give 100% oxygen and ensure adequate lung ventilation (hyperventilation may help by increasing plasma pH in the presence of metabolic acidosis) • Confirm or establish intravenous access • Control seizures: give a benzodiazepine, thiopental or propofol in small incremental doses • Assess cardiovascular status throughout • Consider drawing blood for analysis, but do not delay definitive treatment to do this

3 **Treatment**	**IN CIRCULATORY ARREST** • Start cardiopulmonary resuscitation (CPR) using standard protocols • Manage arrhythmias using the same protocols, recognising that arrhythmias may be very refractory to treatment • Consider the use of cardiopulmonary bypass if available	**WITHOUT CIRCULATORY ARREST** Use conventional therapies to treat: • hypotension, • bradycardia, • tachyarrhythmia
	GIVE INTRAVENOUS LIPID EMULSION (following the regimen overleaf) • Continue CPR throughout treatment with lipid emulsion • Recovery from LA-induced cardiac arrest may take >1 h • Propofol is not a suitable substitute for lipid emulsion • Lidocaine should not be used as an anti-arrhythmic therapy	**CONSIDER INTRAVENOUS LIPID EMULSION** (following the regimen overleaf) • Propofol is not a suitable substitute for lipid emulsion • Lidocaine should not be used as an anti-arrhythmic therapy

4 **Follow-up**	• Arrange safe transfer to a clinical area with appropriate equipment and suitable staff until sustained recovery is achieved
	• Exclude pancreatitis by regular clinical review, including daily amylase or lipase assays for two days
	• Report cases as follows:
	    in the United Kingdom to the National Patient Safety Agency (via www.npsa.nhs.uk)
	    in the Republic of Ireland to the Irish Medicines Board (via www.imb.ie)
	If Lipid has been given, please also report its use to the international registry at www.lipidregistry.org. Details may also be posted at www.lipidrescue.org

Your nearest bag of Lipid Emulsion is kept ....

This guideline is not a standard of medical care. The ultimate judgement with regard to a particular clinical procedure or treatment plan must be made by the clinician in the light of the clinical data presented and the diagnostic and treatment options available.

© The Association of Anaesthetists of Great Britain & Ireland 2010

Reproduced with the kind permission of The Association of Anaesthetists of Great Britain and Ireland

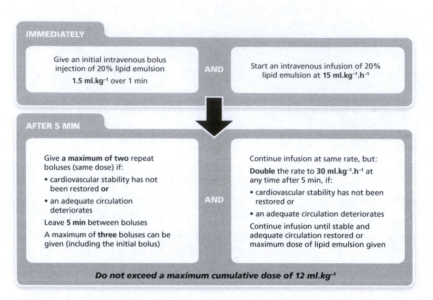

IMMEDIATELY

Give an initial intravenous bolus injection of 20% lipid emulsion **1.5 ml.kg⁻¹ over 1 min**

AND

Start an intravenous infusion of 20% lipid emulsion at **15 ml.kg⁻¹.h⁻¹**

AFTER 5 MIN

Give a **maximum of two** repeat boluses (same dose) if:
- cardiovascular stability has not been restored **or**
- an adequate circulation deteriorates

Leave **5 min** between boluses

A maximum of **three** boluses can be given (including the initial bolus)

AND

Continue infusion at same rate, but:

Double the rate to **30 ml.kg⁻¹.h⁻¹** at any time after 5 min, if:
- cardiovascular stability has not been restored or
- an adequate circulation deteriorates

Continue infusion until stable and adequate circulation restored or maximum dose of lipid emulsion given

Do not exceed a maximum cumulative dose of 12 ml.kg⁻¹

An approximate dose regimen for a 70-kg patient would be as follows:

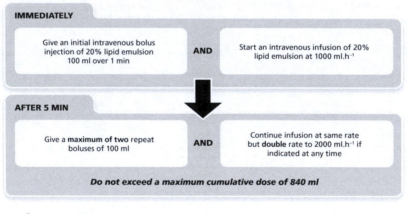

IMMEDIATELY

Give an initial intravenous bolus injection of 20% lipid emulsion 100 ml over 1 min

AND

Start an intravenous infusion of 20% lipid emulsion at 1000 ml.h⁻¹

AFTER 5 MIN

Give a **maximum of two** repeat boluses of 100 ml

AND

Continue infusion at same rate but **double** rate to 2000 ml.h⁻¹ if indicated at any time

Do not exceed a maximum cumulative dose of 840 ml

This AAGBI Safety Guideline was produced by a Working Party that comprised:
Grant Cave, Will Harrop-Griffiths (Chair), Martyn Harvey, Tim Meek, John Picard, Tim Short and Guy Weinberg.

This Safety Guideline is endorsed by the Australian and New Zealand College of Anaesthetists (ANZCA).

Guidelines for the management of a malignant hyperthermia crisis

GUIDELINES FOR THE MANAGEMENT OF A MALIGNANT HYPERTHERMIA CRISIS

The reduction in mortality from Malignant Hyperthermia (MH) is as result of an awareness of MH by anaesthetists, its early detection (diagnosis) and the advances in monitoring standards on which successful management depends.

The mode of presentation of MH varies, and the order of the various modalities of treatment may need to be modified accordingly. The steps below are intended as an "aide memoire".

Know where dantrolene is stored in your theatre.

DIAGNOSIS, CONSIDER MH IF:
1. masseter muscle spasm after suxamethonium
2. unexplained, unexpected tachycardia together with
3. unexplained, unexpected increase in end-tidal CO_2

EARLY MANAGEMENT
1. Withdraw all trigger agents (ie all anaesthetic vapours)
2. Install clean anaesthetic breathing system and hyperventilate
3. Abandon surgery if feasible
4. Give dantrolene IV. 1mg/kg initially and repeat PRN up to 10mg/kg.
5. Measure ABGs, K+ and CK
6. Measure core temperature
7. Surface cooling avoiding vasoconstriction.

INTERMEDIATE MANAGEMENT
1. Control serious arrthymias with ß blockers etc
2. Control hyperkalaemia and metabolic acidosis

LATER MANAGEMENT
1. Clotting screen to detect DIC
2. Take first voided urine sample for myoglobin estimation
3. Observe urine output for developing renal failure
4. Promote diuresis with fluids/mannitol. (20mg dantrolene contains 3g mannitol)
5. Repeat CK at 24hrs

LATE MANAGEMENT
1. Consider other diagnoses and do appropriate investigations eg VMA, thyroid function tests, WCC, CXR.
2. Consider possibility of myopathy, neurological opinion, EMG.
3. Consider possibility of recreational drug injestion (ecstasy)
4. Consider possibility of neuroleptic malignant syndrome
5. Counsel patient and/or their family regarding implications of MH
6. Refer patient to MH Unit

The UK MH Investigation Unit, Academic Unit of Anaesthesia, Clinical Sciences Building, St James's University Hospital Trust, Leeds LS9 7TF 0113 243 3144 Direct line/Answerphone 0113 206 5274. Fax 0113 206 4140 Emergency 'Hotline' 07947 609601 is usually available outside office hours.

This poster is supported by the Association of Anaesthetists of Great Britain and Ireland and the British MH Association.

Reproduced with the kind permission of The Association of Anaesthetists of Great Britain and Ireland

DAS guideline – unanticipated difficult tracheal intubation during rapid sequence induction of anaesthesia in a non-obstetric adult patient

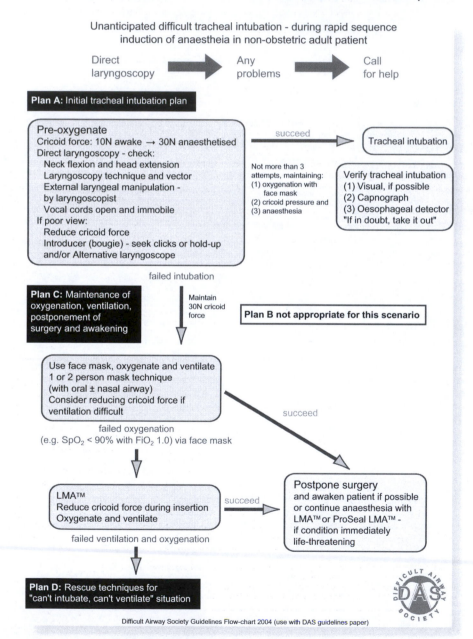

Unanticipated difficult tracheal intubation - during rapid sequence induction of anaestheia in non-obstetric adult patient

Direct laryngoscopy → Any problems → Call for help

Plan A: Initial tracheal intubation plan

Pre-oxygenate
Cricoid force: 10N awake → 30N anaesthetised
Direct laryngoscopy - check:
  Neck flexion and head extension
  Laryngoscopy technique and vector
  External laryngeal manipulation -
  by laryngoscopist
  Vocal cords open and immobile
If poor view:
  Reduce cricoid force
  Introducer (bougie) - seek clicks or hold-up
  and/or Alternative laryngoscope

succeed → Tracheal intubation

Not more than 3 attempts, maintaining:
(1) oxygenation with face mask
(2) cricoid pressure and
(3) anaesthesia

Verify tracheal intubation
(1) Visual, if possible
(2) Capnograph
(3) Oesophageal detector
"If in doubt, take it out"

failed intubation

Plan C: Maintenance of oxygenation, ventilation, postponement of surgery and awakening

Maintain 30N cricoid force

Plan B not appropriate for this scenario

Use face mask, oxygenate and ventilate
1 or 2 person mask technique
(with oral ± nasal airway)
Consider reducing cricoid force if ventilation difficult

succeed

failed oxygenation
(e.g. SpO$_2$ < 90% with FiO$_2$ 1.0) via face mask

LMA™
Reduce cricoid force during insertion
Oxygenate and ventilate

succeed

Postpone surgery
and awaken patient if possible
or continue anaesthesia with
LMA™ or ProSeal LMA™ -
if condition immediately
life-threatening

failed ventilation and oxygenation

Plan D: Rescue techniques for "can't intubate, can't ventilate" situation

Difficult Airway Society Guidelines Flow-chart 2004 (use with DAS guidelines paper)

DAS guideline – can't intubate, can't ventilate

Failed intubation, increasing hypoxaemia and difficult ventilation in the paralysed anaesthetised patient: Rescue techniques for the "can't intubate, can't ventilate" situation

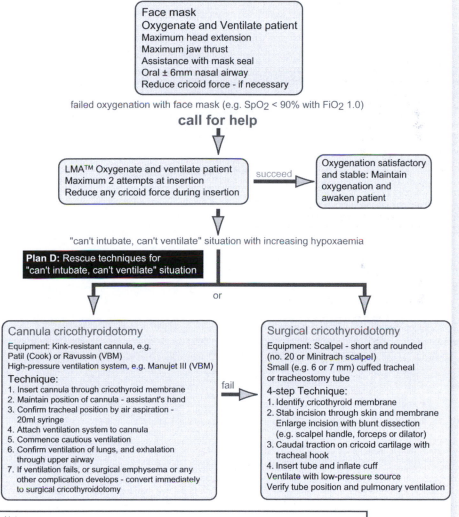

failed intubation and difficult ventilation (other than laryngospasm)

Face mask
Oxygenate and Ventilate patient
Maximum head extension
Maximum jaw thrust
Assistance with mask seal
Oral ± 6mm nasal airway
Reduce cricoid force - if necessary

failed oxygenation with face mask (e.g. SpO_2 < 90% with FiO_2 1.0)

call for help

LMA™ Oxygenate and ventilate patient
Maximum 2 attempts at insertion
Reduce any cricoid force during insertion

succeed →

Oxygenation satisfactory and stable: Maintain oxygenation and awaken patient

"can't intubate, can't ventilate" situation with increasing hypoxaemia

Plan D: Rescue techniques for "can't intubate, can't ventilate" situation

or

Cannula cricothyroidotomy
Equipment: Kink-resistant cannula, e.g.
Patil (Cook) or Ravussin (VBM)
High-pressure ventilation system, e.g. Manujet III (VBM)
Technique:
1. Insert cannula through cricothyroid membrane
2. Maintain position of cannula - assistant's hand
3. Confirm tracheal position by air aspiration - 20ml syringe
4. Attach ventilation system to cannula
5. Commence cautious ventilation
6. Confirm ventilation of lungs, and exhalation through upper airway
7. If ventilation fails, or surgical emphysema or any other complication develops - convert immediately to surgical cricothyroidotomy

fail →

Surgical cricothyroidotomy
Equipment: Scalpel - short and rounded (no. 20 or Minitrach scalpel)
Small (e.g. 6 or 7 mm) cuffed tracheal or tracheostomy tube
4-step Technique:
1. Identify cricothyroid membrane
2. Stab incision through skin and membrane Enlarge incision with blunt dissection (e.g. scalpel handle, forceps or dilator)
3. Caudal traction on cricoid cartilage with tracheal hook
4. Insert tube and inflate cuff
Ventilate with low-pressure source
Verify tube position and pulmonary ventilation

Notes:
1. These techniques can have serious complications - use only in life-threatening situations
2. Convert to definitive airway as soon as possible
3. Postoperative management - see other difficult airway guidelines and flow-charts
4. 4mm cannula with low-pressure ventilation may be successful in patient breathing spontaneously

Difficult Airway Society guidelines Flow-chart 2004 (use with DAS guidelines paper)

Reproduced with the kind permission of The Difficult Airway Society

Index

Entries in **bold** denote boxes, figures and tables.

CPD with Radcliffe

You can now use a selection of our books to achieve CPD (Continuing Professional Development) points through directed reading.

We provide a free online form and downloadable certificate for your appraisal portfolio. Look for the CPD logo and register with us at: www.radcliffehealth.com/cpd

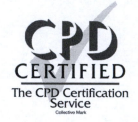